Have a Happy Pregnancy

Teach Yourself®

Have a Happy Pregnancy

Denise Tiran

For UK order enquiries: please contact
Bookpoint Ltd, 130 Milton Park, Abingdon, Oxon OX14 4SB.
Telephone: +44 (0) 1235 827720. Fax: +44 (0) 1235 400454.
Lines are open 09.00–17.00, Monday to Saturday, with a 24-hour
message answering service. Details about our titles and how to
order are available at www.teachyourself.com

For USA order enquiries: please contact McGraw-Hill Customer
Services, PO Box 545, Blacklick, OH 43004-0545, USA.
Telephone: 1-800-722-4726. Fax: 1-614-755-5645.

For Canada order enquiries: please contact McGraw-Hill Ryerson
Ltd, 300 Water St, Whitby, Ontario L1N 9B6, Canada.
Telephone: 905 430 5000. Fax: 905 430 5020.

Long renowned as the authoritative source for self-guided
learning – with more than 50 million copies sold worldwide –
the *Teach Yourself* series includes over 500 titles in the fields of
languages, crafts, hobbies, business, computing and education.

British Library Cataloguing in Publication Data: a catalogue record
for this title is available from the British Library.

Library of Congress Catalog Card Number: on file.

First published in UK 2008 by Hodder Education, part of Hachette
UK, 338 Euston Road, London NW1 3BH.

First published in US 2008 by The McGraw-Hill Companies, Inc.

This edition published 2010.

Previously published as *Teach Yourself Positive Pregnancy*.

The *Teach Yourself* name is a registered trade mark of
Hodder Headline.

Copyright © 2008, 2010 Denise Tiran

Typeset by MPS Limited, A Macmillan Company.

Printed in Great Britain for Hodder Education, an Hachette UK
Company, 338 Euston Road, London NW1 3BH, by CPI Cox &
Wyman, Reading, Berkshire RG1 8EX.

The publisher has used its best endeavours to ensure that the URLs
for external websites referred to in this book are correct and active
at the time of going to press. However, the publisher and the
author have no responsibility for the websites and can make no
guarantee that a site will remain live or that the content will remain
relevant, decent or appropriate.

Hachette UK's policy is to use papers that are natural, renewable
and recyclable products and made from wood grown in sustainable
forests. The logging and manufacturing processes are expected to
conform to the environmental regulations of the country of origin.

Impression number   10 9 8 7 6 5 4 3 2 1
Year   2014 2013 2012 2011 2010

Acknowledgements

I would like to thank Victoria Roddam at Hodder Education for inviting me to write this book and for her editorial support. My thanks also to my friend and colleague, Fiona Mantle, a health visitor and complementary therapy lecturer, for perusing the manuscript and for making many valuable suggestions for the text.

My thanks and love to my partner, Harry, who has endured many months while I completed the manuscript: I hope now we will be able to spend more time together. Finally, as ever, my love and a huge 'thank you' to my wonderful son, Adam, who is the light of my life. Over the last 18 years he has spent many hours 'doing his own thing' while I finished working on numerous books and journal papers and, later, helping me with the vagaries of computer and Internet technology. In the last couple of years he has even taken over some of the cooking and housework so that I could concentrate on my writing.

Adam was born at home after a difficult pregnancy and a long labour. He has, however, been worth every single minute of 'morning sickness' and backache during my pregnancy, every painful contraction throughout a 24-hour labour ending in a forceps delivery (at home!) and every tear I shed with mild depression about a year after his birth. He is now 20, enjoying university in London and eventually plans to work in our beloved Namibia and South Africa. I will miss him when he goes, but I wish him well as he ventures out on his own life journey to Africa and beyond.

Adam is my single most positive achievement, the greatest success of my life: I truly hope your baby will be yours.

Denise Tiran – Director of Expectancy Ltd and visiting lecturer, University of Greenwich.

Contents

Meet the author   xi
Only got a minute?   xiv
Only got five minutes?   xvi
Only got ten minutes?   xviii
Introduction   xxi

Part one – Positive pregnancy
1 **Preparation for pregnancy**   3
    Preconception   3
    Conception   6
2 **Emotions and feelings**   11
    Keep a pregnancy diary   13
    Your partner's feelings   14
    How to achieve the maternity care you would like   16
    Understanding your maternity notes: commonly used
      abbreviations and terms   18
    Dealing with stress   23
    Self-help techniques for dealing with pregnancy stress   25
    Dealing with difficult situations   28
3 **Sex and relationships**   31
    How pregnancy can affect your family relationships   31
    Sex and your relationship with your partner during
      pregnancy   34
    Practicalities of sex in pregnancy   37
    Safe sex in pregnancy   38
4 **Work, rest and play**   41
    Maternity benefits in the UK   43
    Exercising safely in pregnancy   44
    What to do if you cannot sleep   46
5 **Physical well-being**   51
    Physical changes in your body   51
    Eating for a healthy pregnancy   55
    How to achieve a balanced diet   57

Weight gain in pregnancy   63
Things to avoid during pregnancy   65
Some of the antenatal tests and investigations you may
  be offered   67
Beauty tips for self-confidence during pregnancy   70
Coping with physical discomforts   74
Part one: positive pregnancy – the end of the beginning   94

Part two – Positive parturition (childbirth)
6 **Emotions and feelings**   97
  Where to give birth to your baby   99
  Preparation for labour   104
  Packing for labour   105
  Birth planning   106
7 **Sex and relationships**   114
  Choosing who to have with you in labour   115
  Professionals involved in maternity care   119
8 **Work, rest and play**   126
  How your birth supporter can help you   128
9 **Physical well-being**   131
  Powers, passages and passenger   132
  Working with contractions   139
  Conventional methods of relieving labour pain   146
  The power of water   152
  How to cope when things are not as you expect   153
  Induction of labour   154
  Breech presentation   160
  Caesarean section   165
  Part two: happy birthday!   173

Part three – Positive post-natal
10 **Emotions and feelings**   177
  How to approach your new role as a mother   179
  If your baby's birth did not go according to plan 184
11 **Sex and relationships**   187
  Family dynamics   187
  Siblings   188
  Pets and the new baby   189

Family planning 190
Contraception 193
12 Work, rest and play 204
Dealing with visitors 208
Rest and sleep 212
Coping with your crying baby 213
'Time out' for you and your partner 216
Returning to work 218
13 Physical well-being 224
Caring for your perineum after delivery 226
Dealing with post-natal constipation 228
Feeding your baby 229
Post-natal mobility 236
Post-natal exercises 237
Post-natal fitness 239

Part four – Positive complementary therapies
14 Using complementary therapies safely in pregnancy and
childbirth 245
How to take homeopathic remedies in pregnancy 246
Safe use of aromatherapy in pregnancy and childbirth 248
Safe use of herbal remedies in pregnancy 251
Bach flower remedies for pregnancy and childbirth 252
Glossary of complementary therapies 258
Conclusion 261
Taking it further 262
Index 270

Image credits

Meet the author

Welcome to *Have a Happy Pregnancy*!

As a midwife, I have always been keen to help women to adjust to the emotional and physical upheaval that comes with being pregnant. At this stage, the birth seems so far in the future that you probably can't think about it, especially if you are trying to cope with the various unpleasant symptoms of pregnancy, and you may have questions, worries and concerns that need answering.

When I was expecting my son I actually hated being pregnant. I hated the loss of control over my body and the fact that I could not do some of the things I had previously been able to do. I hated the fact that everybody seemed to think I was 'public property' that gave them the right to put their hands on my 'bump' and to ask questions on subjects about which they would never normally enquire. I hated not being able to wear high heels because I had such terrible backache, and that I could not find any maternity clothes which were attractive (particularly underwear!). Even though I was a midwifery lecturer at the time I found it difficult to cope with everyone's assumption that I would know all the answers to numerous questions about my health, yet I had never been in this situation before and could not be objective enough to reassure myself that everything was normal. Of course I had friends and colleagues who were pleased to help me, but I often felt that I couldn't bother them, and occasionally I was too embarrassed to ask. I wished there had been a comprehensive source of information and advice that I could have accessed anonymously at times that were convenient to me.

As a specialist lecturer and practitioner in maternity complementary therapies, I have spent the last 24 years researching the vast range of more natural options available to expectant mothers. Since I had my son, who is now 20, there has been a huge increase in popularity and use of complementary therapies in general, and during pregnancy and birth in particular. Whilst that popularity has expanded the amount of choice for women, the availability of such resources via the Internet has brought with it a degree of confusion, because there is so much conflicting advice which adds to pregnant mothers' bewilderment at a time when they are bombarded by information. The fundamental philosophy in the work that I do is to try to support expectant mothers with both normal midwifery advice and care, and with accurate, comprehensive and safe information about complementary therapies in pregnancy, birth and early parenthood. Any question asked by a mother is an issue of importance to her and to which she deserves an answer which provides her with sufficient information from which she can make some decisions about her health and her maternity care.

In *Have a Happy Pregnancy* I have tried to give you the basics of that information and some suggestions for where you might find additional details, should you require them. Information gives you the confidence to believe in your ability to carry and give birth to your baby and to care for him or her in the early days of parenthood. Gaining confidence will make you more assertive to ask questions when you need, to determine the type of care you feel suits you best and to be a proactive partner in your care, rather than a passive recipient. I hope you enjoy the book and find it useful to help you through your pregnancy.

Only got a minute?

Pregnancy is a time of immense physical, emotional, domestic, social, occupational and financial change, and brings with it many concerns and anxieties as you enter this new phase of your life.

Childbirth is, for most parents, a time of deep satisfaction and reward, with a real sense of achievement. If this is, for you, a time during which you feel unwell or emotionally drained or depressed, keep in mind that pregnancy only lasts nine months. If you are worried and anxious about the birth, remember that labour averages between 12 and 18 hours.

Keep a positive frame of mind and view this period as the 'end of the beginning' – soon you will have your baby in your arms and can begin life as a family.

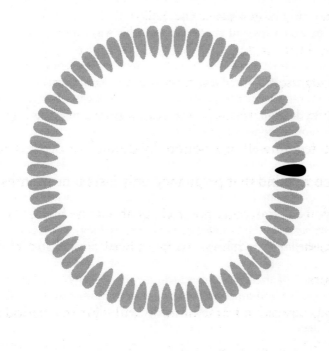

5 Only got five minutes?

The focus of *Have a Happy Pregnancy* is on helping yourself to enjoy your pregnancy, be prepared for the birth and look forward to welcoming your new baby to your family. This requires you to be prepared and to keep as relaxed as possible. Staying relaxed helps your body to function efficiently so that your baby can develop and grow and eventually make his way into the world.

If your stress hormone levels are kept at a low level, your blood pressure will be normal and the oxygen and food being carried through the placenta to your baby will be adequate. You are less likely to develop medical problems in pregnancy and labour and birth should progress normally.

In labour, too, being relaxed suppresses the chemicals which contribute to a greater perception of pain, and this in turn reduces the risks of complications from a long and uncomfortable labour. If your body is able to bear and birth your baby, your recovery will be easier and breastfeeding will be more likely to become established quickly, giving your baby the best possible start in life.

Low levels of stress hormones facilitate the rebalancing of your reproductive hormones and balance your immune system, so you will also be less prone to infections, excessive bleeding and post-natal depression.

Have a Happy Pregnancy helps you to explore ways in which you can stay relaxed, through being informed, asking for advice, communicating with others, considering changes to make your life easier and discovering new ways of dealing with any issue which may arise, including an exploration of complementary therapies and natural remedies. Knowledge is power and, during pregnancy, that means you are in control, even when things don't go quite according to your plans and expectations.

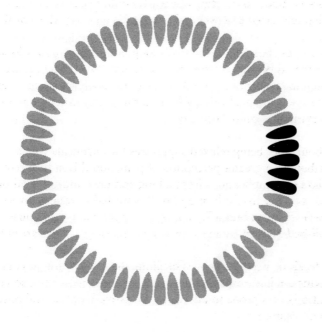

10 Only got ten minutes?

Pregnancy, childbirth and becoming a new parent is a period of immense upheaval. Preparation is key to managing this upheaval during, and even before pregnancy, so that your baby's birth and the early weeks with him are not quite such the shock about which friends may have warned you. If possible, plan your pregnancy by getting as fit and healthy as you can for the three to six months before you would like to conceive, seeking medical advice if necessary. Charitable organizations such as Foresight can also provide preconception care if you wish to look at things in detail.

During pregnancy, ensure that you eat well and, if you can, reduce or cut out factors which may be harmful to you or your baby, such as smoking, alcohol and stress. Take time for yourself and get plenty of fresh air and exercise, rest and sleep: don't push yourself too far. A healthy diet is one in which you eat a range of different nutrients, using foods of all different colours and not over-indulging in any one type of food. Of most importance is the need to drink plenty of fluids. It is not necessary to 'eat for two' during pregnancy, although this is acceptable when you need to produce breast milk to feed your newborn baby.

Work together with your partner or intended birth companion to find out what your options are for antenatal care and for the birth. Don't be afraid to ask questions so that you understand your antenatal care, the tests and investigations and all the advice given by the midwives and doctors. Always remember that you have choices but in order to make informed decisions you need enough information about your options. You may also need to be assertive on occasions if you have particular feelings about what you would like, so it may be wise to take someone with you to your appointments.

Understanding what happens to your body will help you to appreciate the purpose of all those symptoms which can get you down during pregnancy – but if you have any real concerns, talk to your maternity care providers. Pregnancy is a collection of symptoms so do not expect to feel perfect – in fact, feeling the effects of pregnancy means that the hormone levels are sufficiently high to maintain the pregnancy. You may find it useful to explore the variety of complementary therapies and natural remedies which are available to relieve some of these symptoms – but be aware that, just because these remedies are natural, they are not always safe or appropriate in pregnancy. It is best to consult professionals who can give you up-to-date information, based on research evidence, of the aromatherapy oils, herbs and other remedies which are suitable during pregnancy.

Don't panic when you go into labour! If you have planned carefully, everything should be ready and you can relax, knowing that this is precisely what your body is designed for. Most mothers worry about the birth, but the more you can stay calm, the better able your body will be to do its job. Staying relaxed reduces the stress hormones, which helps to increase the labour hormones, and these allow your body to function efficiently so that labour progresses with as few complications as possible and, hopefully, you can achieve a lovely normal birth. If you have medical or pregnancy-related problems and labour is not quite so straightforward, you can still assist the process by using different natural remedies and complementary therapies, but discuss this with your midwife first. There are also, of course, various ways in which the midwives can help to alleviate the pain of labour (the issue that expectant mothers worry about most) – but find out about them in advance so that you can select whatever seems best for you at the time.

Don't have too many preconceived ideas about what you want from your labour and the birth of your baby – things can change very quickly during labour, or you may change your mind about things once you start contracting.

Once your baby is born, it is even more important to be well prepared in order that you can stay calm. Try to get organized during your pregnancy so that you don't have too much to do when you are getting to grips with caring for, and feeding, your new baby. If you are breastfeeding, ask for help from your midwife in the early days so that you can get lactation established: it gets easier as you go on.

Don't worry too much about your baby (although this is very natural) and don't worry about doing the 'right thing'. This is your baby and you will manage – just believe in yourself. Millions of women have done this before you and have felt exactly the same – after all it is nature's way of protecting newborn babies by ensuring that you don't damage them, but babies are actually very strong and children grow up to be adults despite any mistakes you may have made. Remember – you do not have to be 'perfect' – just 'good enough'. Enjoy your baby and relax!

Introduction

Congratulations – you're pregnant!

As you have decided to read this book, you may, by now, be getting used to the idea of being pregnant and becoming a mother, but despite this exciting event you will probably be experiencing many different emotions and feelings – not to mention all those symptoms of pregnancy that you thought everyone else suffered but with which *you* would be able to cope.

Undoubtedly most expectant mothers also have some concerns and worries, perhaps about the birth or being able to look after the baby once he is born – these are quite natural and normal, but sometimes difficult to resolve. You may worry about what is safe during pregnancy, for example, whether it is safe to have that glass of wine or a Brie and cranberry sandwich, if it will harm your developing baby if you take a long-haul flight to an exotic holiday destination or if you should continue mountain biking. You may be wondering about how pregnancy will affect you, your relationship with your partner, your friends and family, especially if you already have children living with you. You will probably find that everyone will tell you something different, often revelling in their own 'scare' stories or repeating 'old wives' tales'.

Pregnancy is a time of immense change for the whole family, physically, mentally and socially, but it is important to focus on maintaining a positive attitude, learning to deal with the issues that can be resolved and to accept and find ways of coping with those which may last until your baby is born, or even beyond. The more prepared you are as you approach labour, the more it will be a positive experience to welcome your baby into the world. And although your new baby will obviously require you to make major adaptations in your life, not least in respect of your social and work life, look on this as a positive move from one 'chapter' of your life to the next. Every step you take towards achieving for yourself and your baby a satisfying – and safe – pregnancy and birth will mean that you are setting your child off on a positive path of his own.

Do remember that this is *your* pregnancy and *your* experience; any choices you make are *your* choices. Being well informed can help you to achieve your aim of a positive pregnancy but try not to become too obsessed with 'doing what's right'. Women have been having babies for thousands of years and the vast majority are born perfectly normal, fit and well, without any complications along the way. Also remember that babies grow into well-adjusted adults because of – or perhaps, despite – the care they receive in childhood. You do not have to be perfect, just 'good enough' to help your baby along the way – and taking a positive approach to the whole experience will help you to put everything into perspective.

About this book

Most books (and much of the conventional maternity services) focus primarily on the physical changes which occur in your body during pregnancy, with everything else appearing to be secondary, implying that your psychological health and your social, relationship, domestic and occupational well-being are less important. However, holistic healthcare recognizes the interaction between body, mind and spirit and the fact that one component of the 'whole' can have a significant bearing on the others. *Have a Happy Pregnancy* takes a holistic approach, exploring not only your physical health, but also your mental and emotional well-being, sex and relationships and how to balance home and work life. It tries to focus on the things that may matter to you, aiming to help you achieve a safe and satisfying experience and a more self-confident approach, in which you can be assertive, ask questions, appreciate the difference between what is normal and what may be a problem and remain in control of your pregnancy and the birth of, and early days with, your new baby.

Have a Happy Pregnancy aims to help you to develop a positive approach to your pregnancy, the birth of your baby and the early days of being a parent by increasing your self-confidence, encouraging you to stay in control and providing a host of practical tips and ideas, including complementary therapies and natural remedies, to facilitate a healthy physical, mental and social outlook.

For ease of writing, the pronoun 'he' has been used to denote the baby. It has also been assumed that the majority of expectant mothers who are in a committed relationship will have a male partner; apology is given unreservedly for any unintentional offence felt by readers who may have different social circumstances.

Part one

Positive pregnancy

1

Preparation for pregnancy

In this chapter you will learn:
- *some of the steps you can take towards planning for a healthy pregnancy*
- *how conception occurs.*

Preconception

Although it is possible that you are already pregnant by the time you read this book, this may not necessarily be the case. If you are considering starting your family, there are some simple steps you can take to ensure that both you and your partner are in good health before conception and for the early weeks of your pregnancy. It is wise, for example, to stop taking the Pill and to use alternative methods of contraception for three to six months before trying to get pregnant, to give your body time to readjust to its normal hormones.

If you are now pregnant, much of the advice pertinent to preparing for conception can also be extended to early pregnancy and, indeed, offers a good framework for family life in the future. Good nutrition is essential to ensure that you have a balance of adequate nutrients and to help reduce the levels of negative chemicals that may be present in your body, either as a result of imbalances in, or intolerances to, your diet, or due to absorption of potentially harmful chemicals from smoking, alcohol, occupational hazards and the environment. Wherever possible, avoid or cut down on refined carbohydrates, excessive sugar, tea, coffee, confectionery and saturated fats and increase your intake of fresh fruit and vegetables. Eat regular meals, avoid dieting and consider multivitamin supplements if appropriate (see also the section on eating well in pregnancy in Chapter 5). Try to avoid or reduce foods that contain preservatives, colourings and artificial sweeteners, especially tartrazine, the orange colouring found in fruit squashes and other foods. Drink at least eight glasses of water each day and give up smoking, alcohol and unnecessary (i.e. recreational) drugs for at least four months before conception. Consider consulting an allergy specialist if you think you may have food intolerances, especially if you suffer from eczema, asthma, migraine, insomnia or depression, which can be caused or worsened by imbalances caused by certain foods. Check with your doctor whether you are immune to rubella (German measles) and if not, ask for a vaccination at least three months before trying to get pregnant, as contact with rubella infection in early pregnancy can be damaging to your developing baby.

Insight

If you are exposed to rubella during early pregnancy, the virus can be passed to your baby, risking deafness (the commonest problem), blindness and heart conditions.

Exposure to hazardous substances can contribute to fertility problems, causing a reduction in the number of healthy sperm produced by your partner or adversely affecting your eggs and hormones. Precautions should also be extended to pregnancy if you are particularly at risk of exposure to harmful substances, for example, because of your job. If at all possible, purchase as much organically grown food as you can afford to avoid the effects of pesticides and insecticides. Other potentially harmful household substances include new carpets and furnishing fabrics, for example flame retarding substances, pets' flea collars, woodworm and dry rot treatment. Avoid prolonged use of electric blankets, microwaves, and any unnecessary X-rays; computer VDUs should be used for no more than three to four hours a day, preferably with a filter screen, and sunbeds should be avoided during the time you are trying to conceive and once you are pregnant.

Certain occupations can bring you or your partner into contact with harmful chemicals, including those in the chemical engineering, petrochemical, printing, decorating, textile and car-manufacturing industries, as well as jobs involving electronic equipment, plastics, battery fluids or nuclear power. Hospital staff exposed to anaesthetic gases and other substances may also be at risk. If you work in one of these areas it is important to take steps to avoid noxious substances, preferably before conception but also during the early months of pregnancy when your baby's major organs are forming – your baby's heart is fully formed within 21 days of conception, so any adverse effects could occur even before you are aware that you are pregnant.

Insight

There is real awareness of occupational hazards these days and much research has been done on how pregnant women and their unborn babies are affected. If you work in a job where you are exposed to harmful substances or difficult working conditions it is even more important to investigate this before you actually conceive so that you can take steps to avoid the risks.

You also need to spend time together as a couple, working on and consolidating your relationship. Pregnancy and parenthood can affect a relationship in many ways and it is wise to tackle any unresolved issues now before you start on this epic life journey. Try talking about how you feel about starting or adding to your family, make sure that you are both happy to go ahead. Is your relationship stable enough to withstand the upheaval that children bring? Look at your finances and consider putting some savings aside. The cost of raising a child until he leaves school is staggering – if we really knew how much it would cost us before we had children many of us would probably decide not to go ahead! If you have any doubts or specific issues in your life at this time perhaps it is wise to delay getting pregnant for a while until you are more certain. If you are having particular difficulties, seek professional help sooner rather than later, whether this is relationship counselling or medical, occupational or financial advice (see the Taking it further section at the back of the book).

> **Insight**
> It may be useful to talk with friends and colleagues who have had children to find out the impact of a new baby on you as a couple, or on the family as a whole if you already have children.

It is especially important to prepare for pregnancy if you have infertility problems, a history of previous miscarriages or complicated pregnancies, if you have any ongoing medical conditions, such as diabetes, thyroid or heart problems, epilepsy, or if you have a higher risk of babies being born with hereditary conditions such as Down's syndrome, for example, if you are over the age of 37. Preconception care is a specialist area of reproductive healthcare, which provides advice, investigations and relevant treatment to couples planning a pregnancy, who may have special medical needs, and your local doctor may be able to refer you to one of these clinics. There are also several voluntary and charitable organizations that offer these services, such as Foresight. You may find *Have a Happy Pregnancy* useful for more information on preconception care.

> **Insight**
> Medical problems can often complicate pregnancy, either adversely affecting your own health further, or causing possible problems for the baby. A medical condition will often worsen in pregnancy or become unstable, e.g. diabetes or epilepsy, although other conditions can sometimes improve e.g. severe skin conditions such as psoriasis.

Conception

It can be helpful, when planning, or in the early stages of your pregnancy, to understand what actually happens when an egg (ovum) is released from your ovary at ovulation and combines with a sperm from your partner (see Figure 1.1). Ovulation normally occurs approximately halfway between two periods if you have a standard menstrual cycle of around 28 days. Some women quite naturally have a menstrual cycle that is longer or shorter than 28 days, in which case ovulation occurs 14 days before the next period. So if you normally have a period every 21 days, which is a week shorter than the standard cycle, the egg is released seven days after the first day of your last period and 14 days before the next period. Conversely, if you only have a period every 32 days, which is four days longer than normal, ovulation – and the possibility of conception – will occur 18 days after your last period and 14 days before the next.

Insight

There is a wide range of what is considered a 'normal' menstrual cycle, but it is helpful if you understand your own cycle so that you can recognize any deviations from usual; keeping a record of your periods in your diary can help to estimate the date your baby may be born.

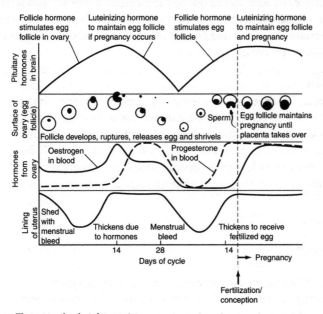

Figure 1.1 The menstrual cycle and conception.

If conception does not occur, your menstrual period will follow, which involves shedding of the lining of the uterus, accompanied by bleeding caused by changing hormone levels (the same hormones that make you feel irritable and bloated before your period). In order for the uterine lining to rebuild in preparation for a possible pregnancy the next month, hormone levels have to increase again and these are produced by the pituitary gland in the brain and by the ovaries. Pituitary hormones stimulate an egg in one of your ovaries to develop and release into the fallopian tube, which joins the ovary to the uterus. If fertilization occurs these same hormones assist in maintaining your pregnancy until the placenta (afterbirth) is big enough to take over this function. The hormones from the ovaries are responsible for building up the uterine lining in the first half of your menstrual cycle and making it suitable to receive the fertilized egg, but if conception does not occur the lining is passed out during menstrual bleeding and the whole cycle starts again.

In order to become pregnant an egg must have been released from the ovary, so the best time to have sex is about 14 days before your next period is due – but allow two to three days either side. If you have been trying for a baby for some time, there can be a sense of desperation around this time and you may want to keep dragging your partner into the bedroom! However, it is not a good idea to have sex too frequently as the quality of your partner's sperm is adversely affected by constantly having to produce semen at ejaculation – in this case, quality is definitely better than quantity.

At the point of conception the egg and sperm combine then start to multiply until there is a clump of cells (which looks rather like a mulberry and is called a morula). During this time the cells have been moving along the fallopian tube and by the time the morula reaches your uterus (about four days after conception) it is mature enough to anchor itself and nestle down snugly into the uterine lining which, under the influence of the hormones, has been thickening and developing a rich supply of blood vessels to nourish the pregnancy. Over the next few weeks the clump of cells differentiates into the embryo (which will eventually grow into your baby), the placenta and the bag of membranes in which your baby is protected inside your uterus. By about ten weeks after conception the placenta has grown and is capable of maintaining the pregnancy by itself, continuing to produce large amounts of hormones to help in the process. It is these hormones that contribute to the many symptoms and discomforts of pregnancy – see Chapter 5. Many of the baby's major organs are already formed by this time, so the remainder of the pregnancy is essentially a waiting game in which the baby develops, grows and matures until he is ready to be born.

Pregnancy is quoted as lasting 280 days or 40 weeks, that is nine calendar months and one week, but bear in mind that there is a wide range of normality, and you may go into normal spontaneous labour any time after 37 weeks, up to 43 weeks of pregnancy. You will be given an approximate date for the birth of your baby, but the length of your cycle will affect the duration of your pregnancy, despite many doctors these days preferring to rely on the dates assessed by your ultrasound scans. It is better to work on the idea that your baby will be born when he is ready, and to give yourself at least three weeks either side of your due date. In this way you will be able to get things organized just in case you start labour earlier than expected, but should not become too anxious (or fed up) if your baby does not arrive exactly on the date you have been given.

Insight

To work out the approximate date when your baby is due, take the first day of your last menstrual period and add seven days, then add nine months. If your cycle is short, deduct the number of days that it differs from the 'standard' 28 days; if it is longer, add the extra days.

E.g. Last period – 25 August + 7 days = 2 September + 9 months: your baby will be born around the 2 June (give or take three weeks).

10 THINGS TO REMEMBER

1 *Keep a record of your menstrual periods in your diary.*

2 *Increase fruit, vegetables and protein foods in your diet.*

3 *Try to reduce salt, sugar, excessive fat and artificial additives in your diet.*

4 *STOP SMOKING!*

5 *Reduce or eliminate alcohol.*

6 *Spend time with your partner and work through any relevant issues.*

7 *Consider the effects of your job on your fertility and chances of conception.*

8 *Check rubella (German measles) immunity.*

9 *Consult your doctor if you have any pre-existing medical conditions.*

10 *Stay calm – keeping relaxed reduces stress hormone levels which can adversely affect your chances of conception.*

2

....

Emotions and feelings

In this chapter you will learn:
- *how to deal with your emotions and feelings in pregnancy*
- *how to plan your maternity care*
- *how to interpret your maternity notes*
- *some self-help tips for dealing with stress in pregnancy*
- *what to think about if you have special difficulties in pregnancy.*

Discovering that you are pregnant can often be quite a surprise, even if you were planning to start a family or to have another baby. It can, of course, be wonderful, especially if you have been trying for a baby for some time, but it also brings with it many unexpected emotions for both you and your partner. You will probably be excited and happy, perhaps even relieved that finally you are pregnant, but you may also feel shocked, anxious, tired, frightened and physically unwell. You may worry about the baby's growth and development during pregnancy; you may feel guilty about what you are (or are not) eating/drinking/doing; you are bound to feel anxious about the birth and how you will cope with the contractions; you may be concerned about how you will cope afterwards, even – or perhaps especially – if you already have other children. All of these thoughts and feelings are quite normal – ask other mothers and they will tell you all the things that they worried about, most of which they will have dealt with better than they imagined.

Of course, finding out that you are pregnant is not something to celebrate for everyone. This may be an unplanned pregnancy; it may be the wrong time in your life; you may have problems in your relationship or you may simply not want a baby. Everyone else will probably be excited at your news yet you do not feel happy, and you may feel guilty about this. On the other hand, even though you want a baby, you may be worried about the pregnancy itself, especially if you have had previous miscarriages or other health problems that could have a bearing on your progress. The hormonal changes will mean that you will certainly be suffering from mood swings and you may keep changing your mind about things, bursting into tears or being irritable to everyone around you. If you have struggled to become pregnant, perhaps needing infertility treatment such as IVF, you will be doubly anxious that everything should go smoothly. Again, all of these emotions are to be expected and most will settle down as you become accustomed to the idea of being pregnant and becoming a mother and as the hormone levels balance out at about 12–14 weeks of pregnancy.

'I looked at the pregnancy test strip and couldn't believe it! Even though we were desperate for a baby, I felt terrified and burst into tears. I didn't tell Steve in case it was wrong and I did three more tests over the next few days, just to be sure. It was almost as if telling him would make it more real than it seemed just by looking at the test strip. Funnily enough, my mother had guessed I was pregnant when she'd seen me the week before – I'm not sure how she knew, she just did.'

Marie, 24, expecting her first baby with partner Steve, 27

It is important at this time to look after yourself – not just physically, but also emotionally. If you can avoid it and are in a position to make choices, try not take on anything that is likely to make you stressed, such as starting a new job or organizing the local school fête. Sometimes, of course, pregnancy seems to occur because you have just moved jobs, had a promotion or moved house and plan to spend money, time and energy on renovating it. But now is not the time to start anything new that is not essential – and if you do have to put energy into a particular task, find ways of getting help.

Asking for help can be one of the hardest things to learn to do when you are pregnant or have a very new baby, especially if you have previously been someone who is totally in control of her own destiny, perhaps with a high-powered career, or someone on whom everyone else relies. Do not feel guilty about asking for help – and if you do, find ways to repay those who help you, if this makes you feel better. This does not necessarily have to be monetary payment but could be something 'in kind' such as minding their house and feeding the cat when they are away or 'house sitting' when they are expecting delivery of a new washing machine. First, try asking someone to do something small for you, such as standing up on the train or bus so you can sit down on your journey to work, or ask someone to carry your bags to the car at the supermarket. Encourage older children to tidy up after themselves, set the table for meals or make you a cup of tea. Ask your partner to stop at the shops on his way home to pick up small items you may have forgotten, or to give you a shoulder massage when you are aching and tired. If you can master these simple requests the more important ones will be easier to make. If you learn now to ask for help when you need it you will find new motherhood a little easier.

Keep a pregnancy diary

It can be useful to jot down how you feel at various stages of pregnancy – indeed, some expectant mothers like to keep a pregnancy diary as a memento of their experiences. It can be interesting, fun and sometimes surprising to look back over this during a subsequent pregnancy. Acknowledging how you feel can be the first step to turning what may initially appear to be negative emotions into positive ones, and can sometimes help you to recognize what you need to do to make yourself feel better. Many of the emotions you are experiencing are due partly to your fluctuating hormone levels – and if they cause that much upheaval, the levels must be high enough to keep your pregnancy going, helping your baby to grow and develop normally.

'When I was about 13 weeks pregnant I felt really miserable – you know, tearful, tired, low and just not wanting to talk to anyone. I didn't remember feeling like that in my last pregnancy with Rich, but when I re-read my diary I realized that I must have felt the same then. It actually gave me hope to think that perhaps by about 20 weeks I might be beginning to feel better – and this pregnancy has been almost a repeat of that one.'

Vicky, mother of Rich and now 37 weeks pregnant

In your pregnancy diary try to identify exactly what you are feeling and then reflect on that emotion and what it might mean. This may help you to decide if you need to do anything to tackle the way you feel, or whether simply having thought about it and written it down in your diary puts the issue into perspective for you. For example, you might feel that you do not really want people at work to know you are pregnant yet, but you are finding it hard to keep from telling them because you feel so sick every morning. Having recognized this, you might then decide to try and change the time that you start and finish work each day so that you can complete your work at a time when you do not feel so unwell, or perhaps you can work from home on occasions. Or maybe you are worried about losing your job: you could contact your local Social Services department for information or speak to someone in your human resources department about maternity rights and benefits. (In the UK it is illegal to dismiss a woman from her job simply because she is pregnant; see p. 265 in Taking it further for Equal Opportunities Commission information on maternity and parental rights.)

Your partner's feelings

Your partner will worry about different things and may not always tell you what he is feeling – he will be concerned about your health (at this early stage he cannot really relate to the baby) and he will worry about money, changing nappies – and sex! Many men find it difficult to talk about their feelings; during pregnancy your partner may give you the impression that he does not care or, if your symptoms (such as constant nausea) continue for some time, he may imply that you should just 'pull yourself together'. This reaction is common, perhaps because men always want to be able to do something to resolve the problem and cannot necessarily empathize with you, since they are not experiencing the same hormonal upheavals. On the other hand, you may want simply to talk about how you feel even though you know it is not always possible to relieve the natural physical discomforts you are experiencing. You could both try keeping a 'pregnancy diary' that you share with each other, which may help you each to see what is important to the other so you can then talk about things together – you might be quite surprised at each other's concerns.

'June's my second wife and this is her first baby so I want it to be OK for her. But I've got two teenage children from my first marriage and I just don't find it as exciting as she does. Also, I'll be 56 when this child starts school and I'm worried I may look a bit like someone's grandfather standing at the school gates at that ripe old age!'

Peter, 51, father of Gill, 13, and Megan, 11, and husband of June, 36

···

Insight

As a general rule, men are 'doers' and women are 'feelers' – they approach problems from different perspectives; this is normal and you both need to recognize the differences and take steps to appreciate the other's point of view.

···

A WAY TO 'BRIDGE THE GAP'

Each evening, try to set aside 20 minutes when you both get home to share what has happened during your day. Take ten minutes – and ten minutes only – to tell your partner about how you feel but also tell him that you do not expect him to do anything about it, you just want him to listen. Then let your partner have ten minutes to tell you about his day and encourage him to tell you about anything that is worrying him. Allow yourselves this time as a therapeutic way of dealing with the changes that occur during pregnancy and early parenthood, whilst recognizing that you both approach problems from a different perspective.

How to achieve the maternity care you would like

At some point you will need to seek professional help and make plans for your ongoing maternity care and the birth of your baby. This can be easy or it may be stressful, depending on what you want and the facilities available to you locally. You may have very definite ideas about where you would like to give birth, either at home, surrounded by family and friends, or in a maternity unit that provides the security of emergency treatment should you need it. In some areas there are also birthing centres, which provide a compromise between the privacy and comfort of your own home and the availability of medical intervention in a large maternity unit, which is usually adjacent to the birth centre (see p. 99 in Part two, Positive parturition, for information to help you decide where to have your baby).

Whatever your decision, you should ideally seek professional advice as early in pregnancy as possible so that any necessary tests and investigations can be performed to ensure that both you and your baby are progressing normally. This is particularly important if you had any medical condition before becoming pregnant, such as diabetes, epilepsy or thyroid problems, if you had problems such as high blood pressure in your last pregnancy or if you suspect you are carrying more than one baby. Similarly, if you have any special social or occupational problems which could have a bearing on your pregnancy, you should consult your doctor or midwife early. For example, if you work in an occupation which exposes you to noxious chemicals, if you are a heavy smoker, if you are an 'older' mother over the age of 35, if you are likely to experience housing difficulties when your baby is born or if you are a victim of domestic violence, it is important to seek appropriate advice and obtain help to ease problems you may have during or immediately after the pregnancy (see Taking it further).

Preparation for antenatal appointments
When preparing for antenatal appointments with your midwife or doctor, write down any questions you may have beforehand so that you will not forget to ask them. Consider taking someone with you who can listen to the answers and act as an objective supporter.

You may need to be quite assertive with your maternity care providers to get what you want and to be actively involved in decision-making, but try not to be confrontational. If you are advised about a course of action on which you do not agree, or which you do not understand, ask for more time to think about things or request a specific appointment with a midwife or doctor who can explain everything and offer opportunities for you to ask as many questions as you need. It can be useful to talk to friends who already have children but avoid listening to anyone who embellishes events and tells you their own 'scare stories'.

Unfortunately, the shortage of staff in many maternity units in the UK in particular, and the excessively heavy workload of many midwives and doctors may mean that, despite attending antenatal care early, you still feel unsure or concerned about some aspects of your pregnancy. Sometimes health professionals are so busy that they 'forget' to give you all the information you need, or alternatively they tell you things in a way that is difficult for you to understand, using technical jargon (see below for an explanation of some of the commonly used pregnancy terms and abbreviations). You will meet many different professionals during your antenatal care but there may be one in particular with whom you feel able to discuss any worries, so ask for an appointment with the one to whom you relate. If you feel that you need to discuss specific concerns or excessive worries there are also professional pregnancy support, counselling and childbirth debriefing services which you can contact by telephone, online or in person, in complete confidence – see Taking it further.

The fact that you are reading this book suggests that it is likely that you want to find out as much as possible about pregnancy and birth, either by reading other books and magazines or through attendance at special classes and events for expectant parents. These can be valuable but you would be wise to find a single source of information with which you feel comfortable – do not, for example, buy all the pregnancy publications in the book store as they will each have a different approach and not all will suit you. It is easy to become confused with apparently conflicting advice, so it is best to wait until you have found one book in which the writing style and clarity appeals to you most.

Understanding your maternity notes: commonly used abbreviations and terms

Most expectant mothers in the UK are given a set of their maternity notes or records to keep for the duration of their pregnancy, until the baby is about four to six weeks old when care passes from the midwife and obstetrician to the health visitor and general practitioner. In other countries you may be given an abbreviated version of your main hospital maternity records. Try to remember to keep your notes with you at all times: in the event of a problem occurring in your pregnancy you can then be seen in any hospital, even if you are in a different town to the one in which you are booked for delivery. However, the notes written by your midwife and/or doctor can often seem unintelligible, especially as they use abbreviations and jargon, and this can sometimes add to any stress you may already be experiencing. Below is an explanation of the most commonly used abbreviations and terms and a brief explanation of each – but if you do not understand anything written in your notes – or about which you hear the staff talking – do ask for further explanations.

For further explanation of some of the antenatal tests and investigations you may be offered, see Chapter 5.

Abbreviation	Meaning
AF	artificial (bottle) feeding
AFP	alpha-fetoprotein test
Alb	albumen – protein, usually in the urine, possibly due to infection
ANC	antenatal clinic
APH	antepartum haemorrhage – bleeding in pregnancy after 24 weeks
ARM	artificial rupture of membranes – speeds up labour
bd	twice daily (usually refers to medicines)
BMI	body mass index – indicates height–weight ratio
BO/BNO	bowels opened/not opened (post-natal notes)
BP	blood pressure
BPD	bi-parietal diameter – measurement across the baby's head
Br / B/F	breastfeeding
CCT	controlled cord traction – method of pulling out placenta after baby is born
Ceph	cephalic – the baby's head – usually indicates position in relation to your pelvis
CPD	cephalopelvic disproportion – your baby's head is bigger than your pelvis so vaginal delivery is difficult
CTG	cardiotocograph(y)
CVS	chorionic villus sampling
Cx	cervix (usually to denote how far dilated in labour)

(Contd)

Abbreviation	Meaning
EBM	expressed breast milk
CV	external cephalic version – method of turning breech baby to head first
EDD	expected date of delivery
ELSCS	elective (planned) Caesarean section
EmLSCS	emergency lower segment Caesarean section
Eng/N/Eng	engaged/not engaged – whether your baby's head has dropped into your pelvis at the end of pregnancy
EPA	examination *per abdomen* – abdominal examination
EPV	examination *per vaginam* – vaginal (internal) examination
ERPC	evacuation of retained products of conception – surgical removal of pieces of placenta left inside after delivery or miscarriage
FBC	full blood count – laboratory examination of blood sample
Fe	iron (ferrous)
FHH(R)	fetal heart heard (regular)
Forc/FD	forceps delivery
Fundus	top of uterus, felt on abdominal examination, used to estimate how many weeks pregnant you appear
G/Gr	gravida – denotes number of times you have been pregnant, e.g. G1 = first pregnancy
GTT	glucose tolerance test
GA	general anaesthetic (unconscious during operation) – rarely used now for Caesareans
Hb	haemoglobin – iron content of blood, should be at least 10.6 gm/dl or above in pregnancy
IM	intramuscular – usually relating to an injection given into muscle

Abbreviation	Meaning
IUCD	intrauterine contraceptive device – contraceptive coil
IUGR	intrauterine growth retardation – the developing baby is smaller than expected for stage of pregnancy
IV/IVI	intravenous/infusion – giving of drugs/fluid (drip) into a vein
LBW	low birth weight – the baby is not as heavy as expected for the stage of pregnancy when born
LFT	liver function tests – special blood tests to check liver working properly
LMP	last menstrual period (first day)
LOA/LOL/ LOP	left occipito anterior/lateral/posterior – denotes position of baby's head in your pelvis – LOA, with the back of the baby's head pointing forwards, is the most favourable for labour
LSCS	lower segment Caesarean section – normal type in which lowest part of uterus is cut
Mec	Meconium – the first black tarry Mecstool passed by your baby; occasionally passed vaginally during labour and may denote fetal distress
MSU	mid stream specimen of urine – clean specimen to test for infection
Multip/ multipara	woman who has had children before
NAD	nothing abnormal detected (on examination/test)
NNU/NICU	neonatal unit/neonatal intensive care unit
Oed/oedema	swelling – usually ankles, legs
OTC	over the counter – medicines you can buy in a pharmacy
P/Para	parity – denotes number of babies previously delivered, e.g. P2 – two babies before this pregnancy
Palp	palpable – denotes how much of the baby's head can be felt above your pubic bone (see Eng/N/Eng)

(Contd)

Abbreviation	Meaning
PIH	pregnancy-induced hypertension – high blood pressure caused by stress of pregnancy
PKU	phenylketonuria – hereditary enzyme deficiency for which all babies are tested a week after birth
PPH	postpartum haemorrhage – abnormal bleeding after delivery (more than 500 ml)
PR	*per rectum* – rectal examination
Primip/ primig	primigravida – woman expecting her first baby
PU/NPU	passed urine/has not passed urine
PV	*per vaginam* – vaginal (internal) examination
qds	four times a day (usually refers to medicines)
Rh	rhesus factor – in blood; blood is either Rh +ve in which rhesus factor is present, or Rh –ve (not present)
SBR	serum bilirubin – blood test taken from a heel prick if the baby is severely jaundiced (yellow)
SCBU	special care baby unit – for ill babies
SPD	symphysis pubis discomfort – pubic pain in pregnancy
SRM	spontaneous rupture of membranes – breaking of the waters
SVD	spontaneous vaginal delivery – normal delivery
tds	three times daily (usually refers to medicines)
Tr	trace – small amount of substance, e.g. amount of protein in a urine sample
TTA/TTO	to take away/to take out – medicines given to take home from hospital
U/S	ultrasound scan
VBAC	vaginal birth after Caesarean section
VE	vaginal examination

Dealing with stress

Some years ago a psychologist, Joan Raphael-Leff, carried out
research into the psychological effects of pregnancy and identified
two types of women, which she called the 'facilitators' and the
'regulators', although it is now recognized that most women
display characteristics of both types. Facilitators are those women
who revel in the very fact of being pregnant, enjoying the attention
and sense of achievement that pregnancy can bring. However, once
the baby is born these women may experience a sense of anti-
climax and sometimes resent the fact that attention is transferred
away from themselves to their babies, possibly increasing the risk
of post-natal depression. Conversely, the regulators are women
who are normally in control of their lives, perhaps having a
fulfilling career as well as running a home; sometimes they are
older women who have left childbirth until later in their lives.
Although their babies may be wanted, these women endure
pregnancy as a means to an end, often fighting against their
physical symptoms, which may make them more prone to antenatal
depression, an increasingly acknowledged phenomenon. However,
after delivery, these women thoroughly enjoy being mothers and
quickly regain control and organization over their lives.

Insight

Some women are not ready to turn their attention to
becoming a new mother until nearer the end of pregnancy, so
may change from being a regulator to a facilitator once they
stop work.

It will depend on the extent to which you are more of a regulator
or a facilitator as to how you respond to normal and any abnormal

pregnancy stresses. Mood swings are common, especially in early pregnancy as your body becomes accustomed to the fluctuating hormone levels, and it is natural to feel a certain level of stress since pregnancy is an event over which you may have less control than you are used to in your everyday home and work life. Some stress is good in that it helps to motivate us to tackle new challenges, but very high levels of stress can make you feel tired and anxious, affect your patterns of eating and sleeping and cause headaches and other discomforts. Continued stress over a long period lowers your body's ability to fight infection and may trigger high blood pressure; in pregnancy, stress exacerbates symptoms such as 'morning sickness' and backache and may increase the risk of miscarriage and pre-eclampsia. In addition, high stress hormone levels interfere with blood flow through the placenta (and therefore your baby's oxygen and food supply), so there is an increased risk that he may be born prematurely and be small and ill. Of course it is impossible to avoid some episodes of acute stress, such as the death of a family member, but if you are dealing with an ongoing stressful situation, for example, a protracted house move, a child's illness, work-related problems or relationship issues, it is important to try to control the effects.

Recognize that this is a stressful time for you but do not allow your feelings to become uppermost in your mind. If you think that things are getting out of control, seek help from your midwife, doctor or, if appropriate, a counsellor (see Taking it further). Being in control will enable you to focus on using your stress positively and may prevent you from becoming overloaded, both mentally and physically. Cut down on habits which you may previously have used to help you overcome the effects of stress, such as drinking excessive amounts of alcohol, smoking heavily or using recreational drugs and try to give yourself time to work things out. Make sure you eat as nourishing a diet as you can, keep hydrated by drinking enough water, get plenty of rest and sleep and try some of the tips that follow.

Self-help techniques for dealing with pregnancy stress

Technique	How to use
Alexander technique	An Alexander technique teacher helps you to learn how to de-stress and to reduce physical effects of stress.
	Can relieve physical symptoms caused by poor posture.
Aromatherapy	Use a maximum of four drops of essential oil in a warm, relaxing bath – lavender, sweet orange, bergamot, mandarin and ylang ylang are safe in pregnancy.
	Do *not* leave vaporizers on for more than 15 minutes at a time and only use oils which are safe in pregnancy.
Bach flower remedies	A normal dose is two drops in water, three or four times a day.
	Use four drops of the Rescue Remedy in water or neat onto your tongue; it can also be dabbed onto your wrists or temples.
Breathing and visualization	Find ten minutes to rest in an armchair or on your bed.
	Take a few deep breaths, focus on exhaling a 'sigh of relief'.

(Contd)

Technique	How to use
	Imagine yourself in a peaceful place such as a beautiful beach, tranquil garden or a favourite holiday destination.
	Focus on taking a trip round your chosen place, continuing to breathe slowly and deeply.
Complementary therapies	Aromatherapy, reflexology, massage and shiatsu are relaxing.
	Always inform your midwife or doctor if you consult a complementary therapist, even if it is only for relaxation.
Exercise	Exercise stimulates your body's 'feel good' (see below) chemicals.
	Drink plenty of water to avoid dehydration.
	Continue regular exercise if you are used to it but always inform your exercise instructor that you are pregnant.
Hypnosis	Buy a self-hypnosis CD if you have specific anxieties, e.g. how to stop smoking in pregnancy or how to prepare for labour.
	Consider consulting a qualified hypnotherapist.
Massage	Ask your partner to massage your back or feet.
	Use a massage glove in the bath to ease your shoulders.
	Gently massage your temples to relieve a headache.
Nutrition	Eat well and regularly – enjoy it but do not over-indulge.
	A very occasional glass of wine for special occasions is acceptable but stop drinking alcohol on a regular basis.
Relaxation	Listen to music, read or simply relax in the bath.

	Have a spa day with a friend (inform staff you are pregnant).
	Spend ten minutes every day doing something you want to do, not something you have to do.
	Avoid situations and people that make you feel stressed.
Stretching exercises	Sit or lie comfortably in an armchair or on your bed.
	Stretch arms and hands to tighten the muscles, hold and relax.
	Repeat this with your legs and feet, pointing your toes upwards.
	Push your shoulders down towards your toes, hold and relax.
	Turn your head from side to side, forwards and backwards.
	Work through each muscle group in your body, stretching, holding and relaxing; remember to breathe slowly and deeply.
Swimming	Go swimming in the day time when the pool is quiet.
	Water-based antenatal classes are good exercise and you can meet other expectant mothers.
T'ai chi or Qi gong	T'ai chi is a gentle rejuvenating exercise, usually taught in classes.
	This improves posture, movement and breathing yet conserves energy so is not tiring.
Yoga	Yoga improves posture, flexibility, muscle tone and breathing.
	Try to find a class specifically for pregnant mothers or tell the teacher you are pregnant.

(See also Taking it further.)

Dealing with difficult situations

Pregnancy can be a particularly difficult time for some women. You may, for example, be worried about being alone with your new baby, perhaps because you do not have a partner, you have unwillingly become pregnant or have chosen to have a baby by yourself, or your relationship with your partner may be difficult or you are exposed to violence at home. Alternatively, you may have an illness or physical condition such as epilepsy, diabetes, deafness, or are confined to a wheelchair, or develop pregnancy complications, which increase your anxieties.

'I was worried that my diabetes would get worse, that I'd have a "hypo" attack and fall over and hurt the baby, but the midwife referred me straight away to talk to the diabetic nurse-consultant about adapting my diet, who also answered lots of my other questions.'

Gerry, 32, diabetic since the age of 13 and expecting her first baby

There are professionals who can advise on these situations but it is not always easy to ask for help, or even to acknowledge to yourself that there are specific issues that are affecting you. On the other hand, significant stress could affect your baby, so think about how you can help him to develop, grow and be born safely, despite your situation. It is not the purpose of this book to cover these issues in depth, but a checklist of specific things about which you may need to give some thought is included here, and you will find some suggestions in the Taking it further section.

What to think about if you have special difficulties in pregnancy

▶ *Have relevant telephone numbers ready to call for immediate support and help.*
▶ *Arrange social support – family, friends, other mothers, voluntary groups.*
▶ *Think about who is going to be with you during the birth and immediately afterwards.*
▶ *Discover how you can meet other new mothers, perhaps those in a similar situation.*
▶ *Consider where you are going to live and with whom.*
▶ *Identify how you will afford/obtain things you need for yourself and the baby.*
▶ *Work out how you will physically manage to care for yourself and your baby.*
▶ *Find out about your rights to financial benefits, housing, childcare and other services.*
▶ *Determine whether the baby's father has any right of access.*
▶ *Identify the rights and role of your baby's grandparents.*
▶ *Make sure you try to find time for yourself.*

10 THINGS TO REMEMBER

1 *It is normal to experience a range of conflicting emotions when you first find out that you are pregnant.*

2 *Take steps to avoid starting any major project at work or home, if possible, to allow yourself the time and energy to come to terms with your pregnancy.*

3 *Ask for help!*

4 *Keep a Pregnancy Diary to record your thoughts and emotions, as well as all the physical things that are happening to your body and to remind you of the things you need to do.*

5 *Try organizing for you and your partner to spend just ten minutes a day discussing the pregnancy and how you feel about it.*

6 *Consult your doctor or local midwife early in your pregnancy so that arrangements can be made for your pregnancy care.*

7 *Write down any questions or concerns you may have and take your list with you to your antenatal appointments.*

8 *Midwives and doctors use a lot of jargon and abbreviations – ask them to explain anything you don't understand.*

9 *Explore ways of keeping relaxed and preventing yourself from becoming too stressed, as this will affect your health and that of your baby.*

10 *If you have particular difficulties during your pregnancy, such as domestic, social, medical or work-related problems, do not be afraid to seek out the various sources of help and advice which exist.*

3

Sex and relationships

In this chapter you will learn:
- *how pregnancy can affect your family relationships*
- *how pregnancy can affect sex and your relationship with your partner*
- *how to deal with the practicalities of sex in pregnancy.*

How pregnancy can affect your family relationships

Pregnancy brings with it potential changes in the dynamics of family relationships, whether it is with your partner, your parents and in-laws or with other children. Deciding when to tell your family, friends and colleagues about your pregnancy will depend on various factors, such as your lifestyle, culture, current relationship with them, geographical distance, your health, previous pregnancy experiences and your occupation. Many women prefer to keep things to themselves until they can be reasonably sure that the pregnancy is well established and the risk of miscarriage has passed, but if you are feeling unwell this can be difficult. There is no 'right time' but you and your partner need to feel happy about your decisions, both regarding timing and exactly what you choose to tell your families. Once you have told them, do not feel pressurized into doing things you and your partner do not want – whether it is about the model of pram to buy, where to have your baby, what names to give him or doing things the way your mother or mother-in-law did when she was pregnant.

If this is not your first baby, or if you have children from a previous relationship living with you, it is important to consider the effects that a new baby may have and how they will respond to the news. It can be very exciting to tell the children about their new brother or sister, but do not be tempted to tell them too early, especially if they are very young – nine months can seem an awfully long time to wait! It is probably wise to delay telling them the news until at least the end of the first trimester (three months) after which time you will have had your scan and may even be able to show them a picture of the baby. You will also hopefully be feeling better than you may have done in the earlier weeks – it would be understandable for a small child to 'blame' the baby for making you feel sick and tired and unable to play. Young children need to be given simple explanations, but be prepared for some awkward questions, both about how the baby came to be 'in Mummy's tummy' and about the impact of the baby on your child's life. Children ask very searching questions, which can sometimes take you by surprise if you are not prepared, but which usually mean that they want an answer. Use simple words that they will understand, do not get too technical and watch out for signs that they have had enough and do not want any more information at present. Your local library or nursery may have some useful, simple books to help with this, such as the excellent *Topsy and Tim: the New Baby* by Jean Adamson (Ladybird 2003). Pre-school children in particular, who may still spend much of their day with you, need to be made aware that this new baby is not going to replace them in your affections. You may need to give them extra attention to make them realize that they are still – and always will be – special. Help them to be involved as much as possible in your pregnancy, feeling the baby move, choosing clothes and toys and possibly helping to think of some names.

Older children also need special care and to be included in the preparations, especially if you are now with a new partner and this is your first child together. Make time and give them opportunities to express any worries and concerns or ask any outstanding questions they may have. If you notice behavioural changes that appear to coincide with telling them the news, try to be patient and not to react negatively by shouting at or punishing them, which will only serve to alienate them. Teenagers in particular can outwardly seem to develop a 'don't care' attitude, but this is often because they care very much, are frightened of being rejected or of getting hurt, or have become aware of their own sexuality and feel embarrassed to be confronted with proof of their parents' sexual activities.

If you have a new partner with children from one or both of your previous relationships, either living with you or with their other parent, you should give some thought to how they may be affected by the news. Their reactions may depend on your individual circumstances, their ages, knowledge of and reactions to the divorce or separation from the other parent, their relationships with their step-parent and any other issues that are occurring in their lives, such as school examinations. You may find *Be a Great Step-Parent* (Hodder Education, 2010) useful if you are in this situation.

'I have two children of my own and two of my husband's from his first marriage. I also had another baby who was stillborn, when I was very ill with serious pre-eclampsia. This really affected my daughter, Beccy, who was 7 at the time – she thought I was going to die, and I am reluctant to let her know too early that I am pregnant again. The problem is, I feel so sick that it's becoming increasingly difficult to hide it, but I'm sure Beccy will worry about me and the baby if she knows.'

Lisa, 44, mother to Beccy, 10, Michael 7, baby Zoe (stillborn) and stepmother to Wendy, 8, and Peter, 5; now 11 weeks pregnant

CASE STUDY

It is also important to think about the impact of your new addition on your family pet, especially cats and dogs – and how you will react to them when you have other priorities. It may be a good idea to identify a place to which your pet can retreat when things become busy, noisy or where he will not be trampled on – and discourage him from sleeping on your bed, even if this has previously been your practice. Both dogs and cats need to become accustomed to different routines, such as no longer relying on set feeding times and to being handled differently, perhaps more roughly than before, once your baby becomes a toddler – but they also deserve some of your time. If your pet shows signs of reacting differently while you are pregnant they may be sensitive to changes occurring within the home. Consider consulting a pet trainer or pet behaviour specialist (see p. 263 of Taking it further).

Sex and your relationship with your partner during pregnancy

Like many parents-to-be, you may have questions about the safety or practicalities of sex in pregnancy but may feel rather embarrassed to ask your midwife or doctor, although they will usually be happy to help or to refer you to someone with more appropriate expertise. Changes in sex drive are normal at this time, both for you and your partner. You may feel less like sex if you are tired, nauseous or uncomfortable, for example if your breasts are tender – or you may want more sex than normal. Abdominal cramping is common after orgasm, but you may feel frightened about the effects of sex on your baby, especially if you have had a previous miscarriage. If these mild contractions continue after sex or you are worried about them, contact your midwife or doctor. If your lack of desire for sex is so overwhelming that it affects your relationship with your partner, consider hypnotherapy or sexual counselling (see Taking it further). On the other hand, some pregnant women enjoy the fact that they can have sex, without their normal birth control method getting in the way or without the fear of getting pregnant when it is not planned. The extra vaginal lubrication and increased pelvic blood supply which occurs naturally usually makes orgasm easier, and some women only experience their first real orgasm once they are pregnant.

Insight

When you have an orgasm it is normal for your uterus to contract and this causes slight contractions. The purpose of these contractions is to suck your partner's sperm in through your cervix (neck of the uterus) and up to the top of the uterus in the hope that, as your egg travels downwards, the two will meet and a conception will occur. Obviously when you are pregnant conception will not normally occur, but you will feel the natural contractions because your uterus is larger and more sensitive than normal.

Insight

There is extra vaginal lubrication during pregnancy due to the hormones; an increased white vaginal discharge is normal but if it changes colour or becomes irritating or develops an unusual odour, it may indicate infection, so check it out with your midwife.

Your partner's attitude to sex may also change. Some men adore the sight of their pregnant wife or girlfriend and he may want to nurture and spoil you. Others find it a big 'turn off' and difficult to reconcile your changing identity from lover to mother, or they become protective and feel overly concerned for your health or worry that sex will harm your baby. However, there is no contact of your partner's penis with your baby, who is enclosed in his own bag of membranes, so normal sex will not cause damage or upset him. He may even be aware that his parents are showing their love for each other and respond to the release of 'feel good' hormones that occur during intercourse and especially during orgasm.

Insight

Sex, especially if you have an orgasm, causes your body to produce endorphins, the 'feel good' chemicals which combat stress hormones. High stress hormone levels can interfere with the production of the positive pregnancy and labour hormones, e.g. oxytocin, so sex can indirectly have a beneficial effect on the progress of your pregnancy.

Some men can feel jealous of the baby growing inside you, or neglected if you do not feel well enough to satisfy their needs. It is extremely important to take steps to overcome this – try to find a compromise, talk about the situation and, if necessary seek professional help. In most cases, if you are in a long-term stable relationship, the problem will pass as your pregnancy progresses. However, if you are not aware of any problems, this can be a warning sign for you (both) to obtain appropriate help. Statistics show that a first pregnancy is the time most likely for a man to have an adulterous affair, and in some men unrelieved sexual tension and the consequent high testosterone levels can lead to violence, which may be directed towards the partner or other children (see Taking it further).

It is important to talk about how you are both feeling and to find the time and opportunity to be together. You do not have to have full penetrative sex if you do not feel like it – just enjoy kissing, cuddling and mutual masturbation. Use music, candles, flowers – even sexual movies if you like them – to put you 'in the mood' and help you feel more relaxed. Massage each other before and during sex with grapeseed oil and two or three drops of essential oil. Ylang ylang is very relaxing and safe in pregnancy but avoid rubbing it in or near your vagina. Add four drops of the oil to your bath and take a dip together, (but do not use essential oils if your membranes have broken prior to labour). Indulge in a romantic dinner or plan a weekend away. Try Bach flower remedies if you are anxious about sex in pregnancy. Rescue Remedy, four drops neat on your tongue, is a good anti-stress remedy immediately before penetration, or try olive or hornbeam, two drops in water, if you are feeling tired (see also Part four).

'We have a very active sex life, but when I got pregnant I just didn't have the energy to keep up with my partner and that started to cause problems between us. At one of my antenatal appointments I met a new midwife who was so lovely that I suddenly started to tell her about our difficulties. I'm so glad I did because she had experience in dealing with this sort of thing and gave me some useful information and sources of help. Just talking to her made me feel better.'

Lesley, 28, expecting her first baby with husband Jim

Practicalities of sex in pregnancy

The physical act of sex can sometimes appear difficult, even impossible at times, particularly as your baby grows larger and you feel more uncomfortable. For example, the increased urge to pass urine in pregnancy can sometimes interfere with sex, possibly being aggravated by penetration. It may be necessary – and even fun – to experiment with various positions during sex. If you are on top of your partner, sitting astride him or on your side, pressure on your 'bump' is reduced, whereas lying flat on your back for too long may make you feel faint.

Lying side by side (spooning) avoids excessively deep penetration and keeps your partner's weight off your abdomen, which can be uncomfortable as pregnancy progresses. Lie on your side curled up, with your partner lying behind you facing your back so that he can enter your vagina from behind. You could also try lying on your sides facing each other; your partner puts one leg over yours and enters your vagina from an angle. Alternatively, you can lie on your back (use a pillow in later pregnancy) with the leg closest to your partner placed over his legs; he lies on his side, facing you and enters you from behind and to the side.

Also use the bed to support you, with your bottom on the edge of the bed and your feet either on the floor or on two chairs placed either side, so that your partner can kneel or stand in front of you. However, in this position penetration can be quite deep so let your partner know if you feel uncomfortable. Try also sitting on his lap while he sits on a (strong!) chair.

Safe sex in pregnancy

Vaginal sex is perfectly safe for most couples in pregnancy. It is, after all, the most natural thing in the world, the point where it all started, so enjoy it and what it means to you both. There are, however, a few occasions when it may be better to avoid sex. During the first three months it is usually advisable to avoid penetrative sex if you have had a previous miscarriage or have a history of abnormal dilatation of the cervix, especially if you have had a stitch inserted to keep your cervix closed. Once you have had your ultrasound scan at around 12–14 weeks of pregnancy, you will know where your placenta (afterbirth) is lying in your uterus. A placenta that is lying abnormally low down (placenta praevia), is possibly the single real reason to avoid penetrative sex during pregnancy as it may cause haemorrhage. In the last three months take care with any sexual activity if you have had a previous premature labour, in particular excessive nipple massage, which can trigger hormone changes leading to contractions. If you are expecting more than one baby, you may also be advised by your obstetrician to avoid sex in the last few weeks, because premature labour is much more common. If you experience any unusual vaginal loss or bleeding during or after sex, contact your midwife or doctor, although a slight brown loss is not uncommon. An increase in the amount of vaginal lubrication is normal in pregnancy but a different colour or unusual odour could indicate infection, which if left untreated could pass to your partner and to your baby.

Insight

Sperm contains hormones which, later in pregnancy, can help push you towards labour. The action of penetration and thrusting during sex can cause a small release of hormones from around your cervix; and orgasm makes your uterus contract. These factors together can theoretically increase the risk of miscarriage if you are particularly sensitive to it, although there is no real evidence to suggest that sex actually does cause miscarriage.

Oral sex is acceptable if this is part of your normal sexual practice but do not let your partner blow air into your vagina as this can cause air bubbles to occur in a blood vessel, which is a potentially fatal problem. Anal intercourse may cause infection and is probably best avoided in pregnancy unless your partner is extremely conscientious about scrupulously washing his penis before changing to your vagina. If you start to develop haemorrhoids (piles), anal sex will, in any case, become too painful and may overstretch the veins in the anus, causing them to prolapse outside. Vibrators are safe if clean and used carefully to avoid damaging the lining of your vagina or cervix or causing infection. Do not use a vibrator in both your vagina and anus without washing it in between. Masturbation can be a very good way of receiving and giving sexual pleasure and is safe, so long as your nails (or your partner's) are clean and short.

If you do not have a regular partner, do not have unprotected sex with someone whose sexual history is unknown to you or who may have a sexually transmitted disease, such as group B streptococcus, genital warts or herpes, chlamydia or HIV. If you become infected, the disease can be passed to your baby, either via the placenta as with chlamydia and HIV, or during labour as the baby passes down the birth canal, as may happen with herpes. Although many women with these infections successfully deliver healthy babies, some diseased infants are born to infected mothers each year, occasionally with fatal consequences.

10 THINGS TO REMEMBER

1   *It is your decision when to tell your family, friends and employer about your pregnancy, so do not feel pressurized to tell them too early unless you want to do so.*

2   *Think carefully, and agree with your partner, about when and how to tell your children about the new baby.*

3   *Talk to your health visitor if you need help to work out how to tell your children, particularly those who are very young.*

4   *Sex in pregnancy is perfectly safe but you may need to avoid it for a while if you have had a previous miscarriage, or if the placenta is very low in your uterus.*

5   *Changes in sex drive are normal for both of you: discuss them and try other ways of showing your love for each other if there is a difference in sex drive between you.*

6   *It is common to have a small amount of dark brown vaginal bleeding after sex in later pregnancy, but if this happens and you are worried consult your midwife or doctor for advice.*

7   *You may need to adapt the ways in which you have sex, experimenting by using different positions so that you are comfortable.*

8   *Take extra care to wash yourself after having sex to avoid the slightly increased risk of infections in the vagina or bladder.*

9   *If your sexual partner has any sexually transmitted infection he should wear a condom when you have sex in pregnancy, to avoid infecting your baby.*

10   *Sex in pregnancy can be a very positive experience, as orgasm releases endorphins, the 'feel good' chemicals which help you to relax and aid sleep.*

4

Work, rest and play

In this chapter you will learn:
- *how to balance your home, work and social life*
- *about considerations regarding your working environment*
- *about maternity benefits in the UK*
- *how to exercise safely in pregnancy*
- *about what to do if you cannot sleep.*

Achieving an appropriate work–life balance is increasingly of concern even when you are not pregnant, but it becomes much more difficult once you conceive and later, when you have had your baby. Of course, for most of us, having a job or career is not only desirable, it is often financially essential and you will probably feel that your priority, especially if this is your first pregnancy, has to be your work. However, it is also important to have time for yourself and your partner, both for necessary tasks at home and in order to take 'time out' from being pregnant, just to be yourself. Many couples try to snatch a holiday or a short break away before the baby is born, especially if it is their first, so that they have had a rest and spent time together, and this may be something you might like to think about if you can afford it.

You need to consider when you will stop working to prepare for the birth of your baby and whether or not you will return to work afterwards. How long you decide to continue working will depend on your health and well-being and the development of any pregnancy complications, as well as the type of work you do, especially if there are specific risk factors such as chemicals or physical exertion. Many mothers choose to work until almost their due date – and may have to do so in order to be able to take off more time once the baby is born. However, this is not ideal. Try to find time for yourself before your baby is born and perhaps do things you may not be able to do afterwards, to prepare for the birth and motherhood – and to rest. You will never, ever have time again to do things totally spontaneously – at least not for the next 20 years!

While you are still at work there are some steps you can take to look after yourself and avoid becoming over-tired. If you sit at a desk take cushions, inflatable pillows and a stool on which to put your feet to make yourself more comfortable. Open the nearest window if possible, or in very hot weather ask for a fan to keep you cool. Work with your shoes off and wear loose comfortable clothing. Take frequent breaks to stretch, walk and go to the toilet. Sip plenty of water throughout the day and avoid too much coffee. If you work at a computer ask for any aids that may make you more comfortable – and to which you are entitled – such as an ergonomic chair and arm-rest for your mouse, and avoid prolonged periods with the VDU switched on unnecessarily. Remember that your employer has a duty to provide all possible services and equipment that may make your workplace more ergonomically and environmentally safe, especially when you are pregnant. You are also, in the UK, entitled to paid time off work to attend antenatal appointments and classes.

Things to consider about your working environment

- ▶ *long working hours*
- ▶ *standing or sitting in one position for long periods of time*
- ▶ *your work station and your posture*
- ▶ *lifting heavy or cumbersome loads, stretching for things from shelves*
- ▶ *working in precarious places such as up ladders or on construction sites*
- ▶ *working on your own, for both security and protection from injury*

▶ *threats of violence in the workplace, e.g. police and emergency service personnel*
▶ *extremes of temperature, noise or pressure, e.g. diving*
▶ *working with chemicals, lead, biological agents or radiation*
▶ *potential exposure to infection*
▶ *working with animals/animal products/contact with excreta*
▶ *jobs which involve a lot of travel or time changes, including shift/night working*
▶ *exposure to other people's smoke*
▶ *dealing with stress and/or discrimination on grounds of pregnancy in the workplace.*

Maternity benefits in the UK

There are many benefits to which pregnant women and new mothers may be entitled. Some of these depend on your income, others such as free dental care, are available for all. For more specific details contact your local Social Services department; the Citizens Advice website has a clear logical summary of all benefits and entitlements – see Taking it further.

▶ *Child benefit – This is a weekly payment to the adult primarily responsible for the child's care, payable for all children up to age 16 (or 19 if still in full-time education). It is not dependent on income or savings.*
▶ *Child tax credit – This payment supports families with children under 16, or under 19 in full-time college (but not university) education. The amount awarded is based on household income.*
▶ *Disability living allowance – This benefit is for physically or mentally disabled children or adults who need help with personal care or who have walking difficulties. It is tax free and not dependent on income or savings.*
▶ *NHS dental care and prescriptions – Free to all pregnant women and for up to one year following delivery and for all children under 16, or under 19 if in full-time education.*

- *Statutory maternity leave and pay – This is a taxable weekly payment to encourage all women to take up to 26 weeks off work before and/or after delivery. You must be employed by the same employer for at least 26 weeks and you must work until at least the fifteenth week before your due date.*
- *Statutory paternity leave and pay – This benefit includes financial payments and up to two weeks' leave to encourage your partner to be involved in the care of your baby. It is based on his income and paid by his employer but he must have worked continuously for the same employer for at least 26 weeks by the twenty-fifth week of your pregnancy.*
- *Sure Start maternity grant – This is a one-off payment from the Social Fund to help those on income support, income based jobseeker's allowance, pension credit or child tax credit with the costs of a new baby. It does not have to be repaid.*
- *Working tax credit – This is payable to 'top up' the low earnings of employed or self-employed adults including those without children, to encourage them to remain in work. It includes extra supplements for families with young children requiring childcare and for those with a disabled family member.*

Exercising safely in pregnancy

Exercise is perfectly safe and acceptable during pregnancy, within certain limits. Moderate exercise has been shown to be beneficial, increasing blood flow through the placenta to your baby and possibly reducing risks of pre-eclampsia and pregnancy diabetes, but excessive exercise can be counter-productive. If you have any medical or pregnancy complications, such as threatened miscarriage or placental bleeding later on, risk of premature labour, high blood pressure or if you are expecting more than one baby, avoid or reduce exercise for the time being and check with your midwife, doctor or instructor about when it is appropriate to resume.

If you are accustomed to regular exercise and remain well, it is safe to continue, albeit with some modifications as you approach the end of your pregnancy. If you attend a regular class, inform your instructor that you are pregnant so that s/he can adapt the exercises as necessary, but it is best to continue with your current programme rather than trying something new which will put stress on different muscle groups. Exercise only until you are slightly out of breath but still able to talk comfortably, otherwise the amount of oxygen reaching your baby will be reduced, even if only temporarily. Do not over-stress or strain yourself. Take care especially with your lower back and with any exercises that require you to place your legs wide apart as this strains your pelvic ligaments and can cause pelvic girdle pain (symphysis pubis discomfort – see Chapter 5). After about 20 weeks of pregnancy avoid exercises which require you to lie flat on the floor for any prolonged period as this can make you feel dizzy and reduces the transfer of oxygen to your baby. Avoid becoming over-heated which can make you feel light-headed and affects your baby's heartbeat; if necessary, slow down or take a rest. It is essential to sip plenty of water throughout your exercise programme to prevent dehydration and maintain your heat balance, especially with aerobic exercise, which should be kept to low-impact work. When running, you may need to slow your pace to a fast walk, and reduce any weights you use in training.

If you are a swimmer, try to keep your spine straight and avoid arching your neck backwards, as can happen if you swim breaststroke with your face out of the water. Dancing can be relaxing and lifts your mood – belly dancing has become increasingly popular for pregnant women. Cycling and horse riding are acceptable if you are experienced but take care not to fall off (even the apparently most docile of horses can occasionally be unpredictable!) and be aware of any adverse effects on your back and pelvic ligaments. Scuba diving, contact sports, potholing, parachuting and skiing are not considered safe during pregnancy. If you attend a sports club that has an on-site spa, it is best to avoid post-exercise saunas as the excessive rise in temperature can make you feel light-headed and occasionally trigger premature labour. Jacuzzis, which usually contain chemicals, should also be avoided and, although whirlpool baths are generally thought to be safe, do not sit directly over the water outlet, as forceful entry of water up your vagina could cause water or bubbles to get into your circulation, with serious, sometimes fatal effects.

> **Insight**
>
> In pregnancy your temperature naturally increases by one degree Celsius because of all the extra tissues and blood vessels you develop in order to help your baby develop and grow. Even a slight additional increase in temperature from exercise, bathing or spas can cause you to become over-heated, similar to a menopausal 'hot flush', which can, in certain circumstances, cause your uterus to become 'irritable' enough to start contracting.

If you have previously done little exercise, now is the time to develop a discipline that will be useful for you and your children. Gentle walking or swimming, walking upstairs instead of taking the lift, exercising the dog or playing in the park with your other children are all easy ways of getting enough exercise to maintain your health and well-being, especially when you are in the fresh air. Pregnancy yoga, pilates and water-based exercises are also good and bring opportunities to meet other expectant mothers.

What to do if you cannot sleep

During pregnancy your body is working extremely hard and it is common to become tired, sometimes to the point of weariness or exhaustion, especially in the early weeks while your body accustoms itself to the massive changes occurring. This will be worse if you are also stressed, as it may be difficult for your mind to 'switch off' when you go to bed, even if you feel ready for sleep. When you do finally get to sleep, you may experience vivid, sometimes unpleasant or worrying dreams, possibly related to subconscious worries. It seems to be a feature of pregnancy to remember more dreams than normal. If you are also physically uncomfortable or need to get up to see to other children, you may also have disturbed nights that add to the problem.

Insight

Tiredness is a normal feature of pregnancy because the hormones exert a 'stress' on your body as your baby starts to develop and grow; the increasing weight to carry around also adds to this – by the end of pregnancy you are carrying an average of 13 kg extra weight.

The amount of sleep you need is individual: you may be able to cope on five hours a night or feel terrible on anything less than ten. If you are getting less sleep than you do normally but are coping, do not waste energy worrying about it. If, however, you cannot cope with day-to-day tasks, see if you can find time to take a daytime nap. If you are at home with small children, rest with your feet up when they have a daytime sleep. At work, it may be difficult to rest in the day but make a conscious effort to move away from your desk at lunch-time, have something to eat and drink and perhaps take a walk in the fresh air – it is as important to ensure that you have enough exercise in the daytime, even if it is only a gentle walk. When you get home, try to eat your evening meal before 7 p.m. and take a short walk afterwards if possible, to aid digestion.

'I thought I'd be all right this time – after all, I've had three babies before – but I was completely shocked by how tired I felt for the first few months. Perhaps it's to do with being that bit older and already having three others. I could hardly manage to cook supper in the evenings, and my social life temporarily became a thing of the past.'

Sarah, 42, mother to Jack 7, Emily 5 and Ben 3; now 34 weeks pregnant

A warm drink before bed may help but your choice will depend on how you feel – for example, you may not want warm milk if it makes you feel nauseous. A cup of camomile tea can be relaxing although not everyone likes the taste – and drinking too much will sometimes have the opposite effect and keep you awake. Avoid coffee, tea, cola and chocolate in the evenings, as well as cheese and wine, which are all stimulating and prevent you from relaxing properly. Many of the stress-relieving strategies we have looked at will also help, including massage, hypnosis CDs and Bach flower remedies. Homeopathic *coffea* – one 30C tablet under your tongue before you go to bed – can be useful if your mind is over-active, you cannot sleep, have vivid dreams or wake up in the middle of the night (typically around 3 a.m.). See also Part four.

Establish a regular bedtime routine incorporating some relaxation – watching the news or a tense movie is not ideal. Listen to music, read a book, try gentle yoga or relaxation exercises, or take a walk around the garden. Make sure your bedroom is warm enough, but not excessively hot, and well ventilated. Lavender aromatherapy oil (*Lavandula angustifola*, or common garden lavender) can be helpful, but use only two drops on a tissue placed on your pillow. If you use a room vaporizer do not leave it switched on for more than ten minutes – turn it off before you go to sleep. Avoid taking anything connected with your work into the bedroom, such as your laptop, and resolve any arguments before turning out the light. Sex – if you feel like it – is a good way of getting to sleep because the endorphins ('feel good' chemicals) that are released help to relax you afterwards and make you sleepy. If you really cannot sleep in the middle of the night, do not panic but get up and have a drink, walk about or read and listen to music. (See also Part three for tips to help you sleep when you are home with your new baby.)

Insight

If you choose to use lavender or chamomile oils to help you sleep, do make sure they are safe to use in pregnancy as there are many different types. If you leave the vaporizer on all night you will continue to inhale the molecules from the vapour and eventually your nasal passages become saturated with them so that you may develop a headache or start to feel nauseous.

Wear earplugs and an eye mask if you are bothered by noise and light and make sure your bed is firm enough – a mattress should be renewed about every seven years to remain firm, but turning it regularly will help (get help to do this during pregnancy). Make sure you are well supported in the most comfortable position. If you have heartburn you may need to sleep propped up on several pillows to avoid regurgitation. If you have backache use pillows to support your legs, your 'bump' and the small of your back. Sleeping flat on your back is not advisable in later pregnancy as the weight of your baby presses on the big blood vessels returning blood to your heart, leading to dizziness, and temporarily reduces the oxygen supply to your baby. Try the 'recovery' position on your side with your upper leg bent across you – but support it underneath with a pillow so that your back is not twisted as your leg pulls down towards the bed.

Insight

In late pregnancy you may need several pillows or cushions to support you in bed, placed wherever your body does not completely rest on the bed – under the small of your back, behind your neck and shoulders, the gap between your knees and the bed. If you are lying on your side, you will need at least one pillow under your top leg, one under your 'bump' in late pregnancy, and possibly one under your breasts if they are very big and tender.

10 THINGS TO REMEMBER

1 *If you are working you may want to talk to your human resources department about your entitlements, including when and how to arrange maternity leave, and any changes required in your working environment e.g. a more supportive chair, reducing duties to less physical ones, etc.*

2 *If you have a job which facilitates flexible working, try changing your start and finishing times, or consider working one day a week at home.*

3 *If you can afford to stop working a few weeks before your due date, take the opportunity to do so: you will not have the time and opportunity again to do things spontaneously until your child is much older.*

4 *Visit the Post Office or search online to find out about the various maternity benefits to which you may be entitled.*

5 *Take time to rest when your body tells you to do so, especially as pregnancy progresses.*

6 *Get some exercise and fresh air each day.*

7 *If you take structured exercise regularly, inform your instructor about your pregnancy so s/he can adapt the exercises for you, or consider going to pregnancy-specific classes.*

8 *While exercising, drink plenty of water and do not allow yourself to go beyond your limits.*

9 *Take regular breaks for a rest during the daytime.*

10 *Take time to 'wind down' before going to bed; do not panic if you can't sleep, but if you become over-tired think about whether you should take a day off work to recoup your energy.*

5

....

Physical well-being

In this chapter you will learn:
- *what physical changes occur in your body during pregnancy*
- *what to eat for a healthy pregnancy*
- *what to avoid during pregnancy*
- *about some of the antenatal tests and investigations you may be offered*
- *beauty tips for self-confidence during pregnancy*
- *self-help tips and natural remedies to relieve physical symptoms of pregnancy.*

Physical changes in your body

Pregnancy is a time of immense physical upheaval and it is sometimes difficult, when you are coping with your day-to-day life at home and work, to remember that the symptoms you are experiencing are necessary and normal. These symptoms are largely due to either the hormones required to maintain the pregnancy and contribute to your baby's development, or to your increasing weight, or both. The earliest symptoms, such as tiredness and sickness, usually start between four to eight weeks after your last menstrual period. By the time you start to feel pregnant your baby will already be three to four weeks old and many of the major organs will be formed, but the hormone levels gradually increase until they peak at about 12–14 weeks, after which time your body is more accustomed to them.

REPRODUCTIVE ORGANS

Your uterus and cervix (neck of the womb) grow to accommodate your baby and there is an increase in local blood vessels and other tissues. You will notice an increase in the normal-coloured vaginal discharge and you may be more prone to infections such as thrush. Although you will not have another menstrual period until your baby is born, you may see a small amount of vaginal blood loss, possibly only lasting about half a day, at the time you would have had a period if you were not pregnant – this is called implantation bleeding and is due to the fertilized egg burrowing into the lining of your uterus. It is normal unless it is bright red or lasts longer than a few hours, but it is wise to inform your midwife or doctor if this occurs, just to be on the safe side.

The placenta is normally attached to the lining near the top of your uterus and provides oxygen and food for your baby, as well as removing waste products and acting as a partial barrier to prevent certain infections and substances from affecting the baby. It produces several hormones including progesterone, which relaxes certain muscles, notably those in your uterus to stop it contracting and expelling the developing baby, but unfortunately it also relaxes muscles and blood vessels elsewhere in your body, producing a variety of unpleasant symptoms.

Insight

Your placenta is the 'power house' for your baby as he develops and grows. It provides oxygen and nourishment, removes waste products from the baby, allows storage of extra energy in case the baby needs it and provides protection from some infections and noxious substances (but not all – some viruses, for example rubella, will pass through from you to your baby).

BREASTS

Your breasts grow (sometimes several bra sizes!) and become very tender as blood vessels and milk cells adapt in readiness for breastfeeding. Make sure you wear a professionally fitted, supportive bra to accommodate your growing size and prevent muscle strain and backache. Of course, some women think it is wonderful to have voluptuous breasts! Colostrum, a thin fluid which precedes milk production, is present in the breasts from about 16 weeks of pregnancy to clear the ducts in preparation for breastfeeding. This may leak from your nipples in later weeks, so you may wish to wear breast pads to prevent it from staining your outer clothes.

Insight

Colostrum helps to clear the milk ducts in readiness for lactation and is the thin, but highly nutritious liquid which provides your baby with his first feed after birth.

'One of the worst things about my pregnancy was how uncomfortable my breasts became as they got heavier. They started to cause pain between my shoulders and ribs, as well as heartburn, and I couldn't bear my boyfriend touching them in the first few months. Then I was fitted for one of those awful maternity bras and my back felt much better.'

Maddy, 25, first baby

CASE STUDY

CIRCULATION

There is an increased amount of blood circulating round your body in order to provide food and oxygen for your baby via the placenta, and your temperature and heart rate increase accordingly. Interestingly, your blood pressure normally goes down in the middle of pregnancy, despite the extra blood supply, because progesterone relaxes the blood vessel walls, so blood flows through under less pressure. A slight increase towards the end of pregnancy is normal, but high blood pressure can lead to pre-eclampsia, which presents some risks to both you and your baby. Swelling of your ankles, fingers and face is common in late pregnancy but if you also have high blood pressure this can be a sign of pre-eclampsia.

Cramp is another common irritation in pregnancy, possibly due to changes in your circulation and salt levels in your blood.

DIGESTIVE SYSTEM

Your sense of taste changes and you may go off foods and drinks you previously enjoyed, or you may suddenly start craving unusual foods, thought to indicate a deficiency of specific nutrients, for example the strange desire to eat coal may signify a lack of carbon in your body. You may not feel very much like eating, especially if you are nauseous, or conversely you may develop a voracious appetite. Some mothers have a peculiar taste in the mouth, often described as bitter or metallic, while others experience an increase in saliva. Constipation, heartburn and haemorrhoids (piles) are common because of the progesterone relaxing your intestines (gut), while oestrogen, and other hormones such as thyroid hormone, are the main culprits that cause nausea and vomiting.

Insight

Progesterone is the hormone responsible for most of the discomforts of pregnancy because it relaxes a certain type of muscle. The purpose of progesterone is to stop your uterus contracting, causing miscarriage or premature labour, but it also relaxes other parts of your body, causing varicose veins in your legs and vulva, haemorrhoids (piles), heartburn from relaxation of the valve at the top of your stomach, backache from relaxation of joints and ligaments and several other symptoms.

URINARY SYSTEM

Pressure from your growing uterus in early pregnancy and from your baby's head as it drops down into your pelvis before labour will make you feel as if you constantly need to urinate. Urinary infections are more common because relaxation of the ureters, the tubes leading from your kidneys to the bladder, causes 'kinking', much like an over-stretched piece of elastic; small pools of urine collect in the 'kinked' tubes, which can then become infected.

54

The relaxing effects of progesterone on your pelvic floor muscles can also cause slight leakage of urine when you cough or laugh – now is the time to start those life-long pelvic floor exercises.

SKELETON

As your baby grows, your weight and abdominal size increase, and the resulting pressure contributes to backache and, occasionally, sciatica (pain down your legs from nerve pressure). Stretching of the ligaments in your pelvis causes groin pain and various unexplained aches and discomforts. If your breasts become excessively heavy, this will put pressure on your upper spine and you may experience pain between your shoulder blades. This can be partly relieved by wearing a well-supporting maternity bra.

Think of all these changes as an indication that your pregnancy is established and your baby is growing, although it is sometimes difficult to cope with them (see below for self-help tips and natural remedies). More excitingly, you should normally start to feel your baby moving at around 22 weeks of pregnancy if this is your first baby, and a little earlier, perhaps 18–20 weeks, if this is your second or subsequent baby. It is often described initially as feeling like eyelashes gently flickering against your insides and at first you may not realize what it is, but eventually as your baby becomes bigger and stronger you will feel periodic movements and kicks throughout the day. This can make your pregnancy feel 'real' at last and help you to realize that all those unpleasant symptoms are due to your baby growing inside you.

Eating for a healthy pregnancy

Healthy development and growth of your baby and maintenance of your own health is dependent on eating well before and during pregnancy, but 'eating well' does not mean 'eating for two'. It is very true that 'you are what you eat'. Health is affected not only by the quality and quantity of food eaten but also by your body's ability to absorb, digest and use the nutrients in food. We each have unique nutritional requirements but these change at times such as puberty, prior to a period, before and during pregnancy and breastfeeding and as you approach menopause. Inherited factors, stress and your general health will also affect your pregnancy nutrition requirements. Food quality can be affected by poor soil, use of pesticides, manufacture and storage, addition of preservatives and colourings, as well as by cooking methods. In today's fast-paced life, changes in shopping practices, storage and types of food eaten, as well as the trend for eating highly processed, ready-prepared and 'fast' foods, often containing little essential nutrients, all affect our health. Drinking too much tea, coffee, alcohol and cola drinks may lead to reduced absorption of essential nutrients, while increased sensitivity to certain foods, particularly wheat or dairy products, can affect health in small ways which are not always apparent. Environmental toxins and pollutants, nicotine, prescribed (or recreational) drugs, plus your individual constitution may also lead to poor nutrition, even though you may be eating sufficient quantities of the 'right' foods.

Good nutrition helps you even before pregnancy by ensuring your body is able to conceive and maintain the fertilized egg. Later, it helps to avoid your baby developing conditions caused by inadequate vitamins, minerals or other essential nutrients. Infertility, recurrent miscarriage and birth defects can be associated with poor nutrition, and smoking and excessive caffeine intake will increase this risk. It is not necessary to take vitamin and mineral supplements routinely during pregnancy, although in the UK, folic acid is advised for three to six months before conception and for the first 12 weeks of pregnancy to prevent spinal defects in your baby, such as spina bifida. Iron tablets are not given routinely during pregnancy but if you become anaemic you may be prescribed them.

You can take steps to achieve a healthy pregnancy by eating a balance of foods from all the different food groups, and generally cutting down on animal fats, salt, sugar, stimulants, processed foods and those with additives and preservatives. Try to increase the amount of fresh fruit and vegetables to at least five portions a day – this might be a glass of fresh orange juice with your breakfast, a banana mid-morning, a salad with your sandwich at lunch, green vegetables with supper, followed by a piece of fruit. You should also drink at least eight glasses of water a day – if you find it difficult to remember to drink water, keep a bottle on your desk while at work. At home, keep a small glass by the kitchen sink and every time you go into the kitchen, drink a glassful – you will soon have consumed the required amount. Cut down on tea, coffee, cola and, of course, alcohol. Current UK guidelines suggest complete avoidance of alcohol during pregnancy, except for the very occasional glass of wine for a special event. If you drink tea and/or coffee, even in moderation, drink one glass of water for every cup of beverage in addition to your eight required glasses.

How to achieve a balanced diet

The best idea is 'all things in moderation'. Avoid going overboard on any one type of food: even 'good' foods can be harmful if eaten in excess. Try to include a little of each type of food in the groups below – use the chart to help you devise interesting and nutritious meals for you and your family. Also aim to have a diet that is varied. Plan meals using different coloured foods, e.g. a salad of green lettuce and cucumber, yellow peppers, red tomatoes, orange carrots, purple beetroot, brown mushrooms and white asparagus. This not only makes a meal more appetizing but also provides a wide range of essential nutrients. See also Things to avoid during pregnancy later in this chapter.

Nutrients and their functions	Where you will find them	Comments
Proteins are needed for growth/ development of blood cells, hormones and other chemicals, for antibodies to fight infection, for wound healing and to produce haemoglobin to carry oxygen round your body.	Proteins are found in meat, poultry, fish, cereals, cheese, milk, beans, peas, soy products, buck wheat, millet, artichokes, beetroot, aubergine (eggplant), courgettes (zucchini), nuts and seeds.	Cook meat properly. Avoid soft cheese, e.g. Brie – may contain bacteria which cause listeria infection. Vitamin B_6 is needed for proper digestion (see below).
Essential fatty acids are required for energy, heat insulation and normal body function, vitamin and calcium absorption. Poly-unsaturated fatty acids are best – they are readily converted to energy. A balance of each type is required.	Unsaturated fatty acids are found in fish oils and vegetable oils, especially safflower and sunflower, (but not coconut and palm oil). Saturated fats are found in butter, meat fat and margarine.	Digestion of essential fatty acids relies on minerals such as zinc, magnesium, selenium, vitamins B_3, C and E (see below).
Carbohydrates are needed for energy, to regulate digestion and keep a balance between normal healthy bacteria and undesirable bacteria that cause infections.	Carbohydrates are found in sugar, fruit and 'hidden' in savoury foods, e.g. tomato ketchup, baked beans, bread, pasta, flour, cereals, potatoes, bananas, beetroot, dates, figs, maple syrup, etc.	Ideally, carbohydrates should comprise 25–30% of total food intake in pregnancy.

Nutrients and their functions	Where you will find them	Comments
Vitamin A is needed for growth and repair of cells, to fight infection, for protein digestion and removal of toxins by the liver, and for healthy eyes, especially night vision.	Good sources of vitamin A include liver, kidneys, eggs and dairy produce, apricots, carrots, broccoli, parsley, yellow and green leafy vegetables and fish oils.	Avoid excessive coffee or alcohol consumption which interfere with absorption of vitamin A.
Vitamin B_1 (thiamin) maintains nerves, heart muscle and digestive tissues, aids carbohydrate digestion.	Vitamins B_1 and B_2 are found in whole grains, nuts, seeds, brewer's yeast, green vegetables, liver, kidneys, fish, eggs and milk.	Stress, alcohol, coffee, preservatives, excess sugar consumption and over cooked vegetables affect B_1 absorption.
Vitamin B_2 (riboflavin) aids digestion of fats, proteins and carbohydrates, promotes wound healing, hormone regulation and growth and development of your baby.		The contraceptive Pill and strong antibiotics affect B_2 absorption.
Vitamin B_3 (niacin) converts food to energy, aids digestion of fats, proteins and carbohydrates, and regulates hormones and other chemicals.	B_3 is found in lean meat, poultry, fish, liver, grains, yeast and butter.	Alcohol, stress, coffee, eating lots of carbohydrates and some strong antibiotics affect B_3 absorption.

(Contd)

Nutrients and their functions	Where you will find them	Comments
Vitamin B$_6$ (pyridoxine) is needed for protein digestion, production of antibodies, for red blood cells, healthy teeth and the development of the nervous system.	Good sources of B$_6$ include bananas, grapefruit, prunes and raisins as well as foods containing other B vitamins.	You need B$_6$ in pregnancy to prevent 'morning sickness', anaemia, depression and skin irritation.
Vitamin B$_{12}$ (cobalamin) is important for bone marrow, red blood cells, the nervous system, cell formation and carbohydrate digestion.	B$_{12}$ is found in liver, kidney, fish and shellfish, (but avoid too much shellfish in pregnancy as levels of another mineral, cadmium, can affect absorption of more beneficial minerals).	Vegetarian diet, epilepsy, the contraceptive Pill, aspirin and codeine may affect proper absorption. Deficiency causes a type of anaemia, poor growth, memory loss and nervous disorders.
Folic acid is needed for blood cells and body chemicals, nervous and digestive system functioning. It is essential for the development of your baby's spine.	Leafy greens, whole grains and some cereals, nuts, oranges, broccoli, tuna, liver and kidney all contain good sources of folic acid.	Alcohol, stress, aspirin, some strong anti-infection or epilepsy drugs affect absorption.

Nutrients and their functions	Where you will find them	Comments
Vitamin C is essential for cells, tissues, nerves, teeth and bone health, wound healing and iron absorption.	Vitamin C is found in oranges, lemons, limes, grapefruit, tangerines, blackberries, blackcurrants, melons, tomatoes, potatoes, parsley and green vegetables.	Aspirin, antibiotics, steroids, the contraceptive Pill and antidepressants interfere with absorption, as do excess tea drinking, pollution and overcooked or poorly stored food.
Vitamin D helps absorption of calcium for healthy bones and teeth. It is needed for blood clotting, kidneys, the heart and nervous system.	The main source of vitamin D is the sunshine, but it is also found in fish liver oils, liver, brewer's yeast, tuna and avocados.	Drugs such as laxatives for constipation and antacids for heartburn will affect absorption.
Vitamin E maintains major bodily functions, including reproduction. It helps your body to respond to stress (and slows down the ageing process).	Vitamin E is found in whole grains, eggs, leafy greens, broccoli, cabbage, avocados, nuts, liver, kidneys and cold-pressed vegetable oils.	The contraceptive Pill and thyroid hormones affect absorption. Food processing and rancid fats destroy vitamin E.

(Contd)

Nutrients and their functions	Where you will find them	Comments
Calcium is important for bones and teeth, blood clotting and to regulate heart rhythm. In pregnancy it is known to prevent or reduce the severity of pre-eclampsia (high blood pressure).	Good sources of calcium include milk, yogurt, egg yolk, sardine bones and salmon, green beans, bone marrow, tofu and soya beans. (It is not necessary to drink extra milk in pregnancy if you eat other dairy produce.)	A high protein diet, stress, too much or too little exercise, antacids, laxatives, diuretic drugs for fluid retention and epilepsy drugs affect absorption.
Zinc is essential for the brain, thyroid, liver, kidneys, lungs, growth of skeleton, skin and hair, wound healing and other body functions. Calcium, copper, vitamins A, B_6, B_{12} and C are needed for zinc absorption.	Herrings, oysters, fish bones, liver, red meat and bones, eggs, milk, nuts, whole grains, mushrooms, leafy green vegetables and paprika are all good sources of zinc.	Tea, coffee, alcohol, processed grains, iron tablets and bran affect absorption of zinc. Heavy sweating and stress also cause zinc to be passed out in your urine.
Iron is important for red blood cells to transport oxygen round the body, bone growth, disease resistance and protein digestion.	Iron is found in red meat, liver, sardines, eggs, wholemeal bread, cereal, chapatis, oatcakes, potatoes, parsley, chives, spinach, dried fruits, nuts, cherries, soya beans, red kidney beans, lentils and chick peas.	Low iron levels cause anaemia, tiredness, headaches, palpitations and heartburn. Absorption is helped by drinking orange juice but adversely affected by tea and coffee consumption.

Weight gain in pregnancy

Normal pregnancy weight gain is between 11 and 16 kilograms (25–35 lb), although midwives and doctors are less concerned these days with monitoring your weight than was the case a few years ago. An increase in weight is due not only to your growing baby and the surrounding fluid and placenta but also to the development of additional body tissues to support growth and development and to prepare you for labour and breastfeeding. By the end of pregnancy the approximate distribution of extra weight is about 3.5 kg for your baby, 2 kg for the placenta and extra fluid and 1 kg for the extra muscles and blood vessels in the uterus, with about 4–5 kg for extra fat tissue all over your body. It is estimated that even your breasts gain about 1.5 kg!

Dieting to lose weight is not recommended during pregnancy, even for those who are overweight, unless it is done under the supervision of a dietician. Some women worry about how much weight they are gaining – sadly, some teenagers even take up smoking as they have heard that the baby will be smaller and therefore the birth will be easier, but it is well known that smoking can make your baby ill, and premature birth is a very real possibility. Unfortunately, the publicity surrounding 'celebrity pregnancies' does not help those of us who are 'mere mortals' as we strive to emulate their consciously restricted antenatal weight gain and post-natal weight loss. It could, of course, simply be a particular design of clothing, a flattering angle of the camera or an airbrushed photograph that appears to make them remain slender and beautiful, but it may be reassuring to know that celebrities have as many weight and beauty worries during pregnancy as the rest of us, perhaps even more so when there is such an expectation that they will adhere to our 'ideal' image. On the other hand, putting on too much weight can make you very tired and increase the risk of backache, swollen ankles, high blood pressure and long-term obesity. Sometimes, however, weight gain can be due to fluid retention, excessive water around your baby or twins, so if you have any worries, talk to your midwife or doctor.

If you are unable to eat a nourishing diet because you are nauseous,
have heartburn or simply feel too unwell to eat, do not worry –
your body will catch up on what it needs when you feel better. Do
not feel guilty about what you are, or are not, eating – this will just
make you feel worse. It is, however, essential that you always try
to drink plenty of water throughout the day. If you have previously
eaten mainly highly processed, ready-prepared or fast food, now
is a good time to think about how you might change your eating
habits. This is something that you can do for your baby – and if
you try to develop new habits now you will be able to apply them
to your new family, ensuring that your child grows up as healthy
and fit as possible. If you feel that you need help, ask to speak to
one of the dieticians in your local maternity unit – your midwife
should be able to refer you. If you need help to break the habit
of overeating, why not consider hypnosis? Several good CDs are
available to assist with eating problems. If you are on a low income
or receiving state benefits, you may be entitled to financial help,
perhaps in the form of food vouchers and milk coupons to ensure
that you are able to buy inexpensive nutritious foods essential for
your growing baby. In the UK, Sure Start, a government initiative
to help disadvantaged families and specific local communities, may
be able to put you in touch with a variety of services and sources of
help (see Taking it further).

Things to avoid during pregnancy

Everyone will tell you there are things you should and should not be doing while you are pregnant, because it is 'bad' for you or for your baby. There are certain things that are best avoided, including some foods and certain drugs and medicines, which are known to be detrimental while your baby is developing. Some foods are more prone to harbour harmful bacteria so should be avoided, or cooked very thoroughly before eating, while others contain potentially harmful chemicals. Some drugs that you may require for an existing medical condition need to be modified when planning a pregnancy or once you are pregnant, while others should be avoided during the early months but may be acceptable later on. However, if you have any doubts, avoid them until you can find out how they may affect you or your baby, or talk to your midwife or doctor about your concerns.

FOODS TO AVOID DURING PREGNANCY

▶ *soft cheese, e.g. Brie, Camembert, certain goats' cheese and blue cheeses, e.g. Danish Blue, made with a mould which may contain potentially harmful listeria bacteria*
▶ *patés (meat, poultry and vegetable) which can also contain listeria*
▶ *raw and rare meat such as steak tartare, barbecued meat, especially sausages, burgers and chicken, which may contain bacteria that cause food poisoning*
▶ *raw and partially cooked eggs, as in mayonnaise and lightly cooked omelettes, which may contain salmonella, which causes food poisoning*
▶ *liver and liver products, e.g. paté, to avoid excessively high levels of vitamin A, which can harm your baby*
▶ *certain types of fish, e.g. tuna (fresh and tinned), shark and marlin, which may contain high levels of mercury, which is capable of damaging your baby's nervous system*
▶ *raw shellfish can cause food poisoning and affect absorption of essential minerals*

- *peanuts and nut products if you, your partner or a close family member has a nut allergy or other allergic conditions such as hay fever, eczema or asthma*
- *alcohol, tea, coffee and cola as research suggests that excessive amounts of caffeine can result in low birth weight babies and occasionally miscarriage.*

DRUGS TO AVOID IN PREGNANCY

- *recreational drugs such as cocaine, crack, heroin, methamphetamine, marijuana*
- *cigarettes and other tobacco and inhaled substances*
- *alcohol, except a very occasional small drink on special occasions*
- *X-rays and radiological investigations*
- *aspirin, iboprufen and other non-steroidal anti-inflammatory drugs*
- *paracetamol, except very occasionally as per prescription*
- *strong laxatives such as senna to treat constipation*
- *decongestants for colds and flu, especially those containing ephedrine*
- *several cough medicines – check with your pharmacist*
- *over-the-counter remedies for cystitis, which may contain high salt levels*
- *antihistamines for hayfever, except on the advice of your doctor*
- *anticoagulants (blood thinning drugs) unless prescribed by your doctor*
- *certain anti-depressant drugs*
- *very strong antibiotics such as tetracycline and chloramphenicol*
- *some drugs used for serious skin disorders such as acne or psoriasis*
- *drugs for medical conditions, e.g. epilepsy, diabetes may need to be changed*
- *herbal medicines and oils, e.g. St John's wort, black or blue cohosh, basil, sage (see also Part four).*

Insight

If you are prescribed drugs by your doctor, only those which are considered safe enough to take in pregnancy will be prescribed – they are not allowed to prescribe those known to cause problems for your developing baby, and you need to balance the very slight risk to your baby and taking something which your doctor feels is needed, with the greater risk to you or your baby if a medical problem such as an infection is left untreated.

Some of the antenatal tests and investigations you may be offered

Below is a brief summary of the main tests and investigations that may be offered during your pregnancy. Some of these are routine, while others will only be offered in special circumstances. In order to stay in control, it may help if you understand why the different tests are offered and that you have a choice whether to have them or not. More comprehensive information and explanation about individual tests, to help you to make well-informed decisions, can be found on the Antenatal Results and Choices (ARC) website – see Taking it further.

Test	Reason for test
alphafeto protein (AFP)	This is a blood test to detect spina bifida, Down's syndrome and other abnormalities in the baby. It is usually carried out at 16 weeks of pregnancy.
amniocentesis	This involves the removal of some fluid surrounding the baby, at about 16 weeks of pregnancy to test for hereditary diseases, or, in later pregnancy, occasionally to remove excessive fluid (not routine).

(Contd)

Test	Reason for test
booking blood tests	Blood samples are taken at your first antenatal appointment to check your blood group, rhesus factor, iron level, immunity to German measles and for the presence of certain infections.
cardiotocography (CTG)	The electronic monitoring of your baby's heart (*cardio-*) and how he responds to any uterine contractions (*-toco-*) you may be having and shown on a monitor (*-graphy*). This is usually monitored via transducers placed on your abdomen. Sometimes in labour your baby's heart rate may be monitored via an electrode placed on his head during an internal examination.
chorionic villus sampling (CVS)	This procedure is performed after 11 weeks of pregnancy (i.e. earlier than amniocentesis) to test small samples of placenta to examine the baby's DNA for hereditary conditions. Usually you have an ultrasound scan to help locate your placenta. There is a very small risk (one per cent) of miscarriage from the procedure (not routine).
cordocentesis	This test is performed after 18 weeks of pregnancy to obtain a sample of the baby's blood for testing, although it is less used now other tests (e.g. amniocentesis) are available. It can also be used to give the baby a blood transfusion while still in the uterus (not routine).

Test	Reason for test
glucose tolerance test (GTT)	This is a blood and urine test to identify pregnancy diabetes. You are given a strong glucose drink and then asked to provide blood and urine samples regularly over the next few hours. It is usually done in response to a routine urine test showing the presence of sugars, although this does not always indicate diabetes (not routine but quite common).
nuchal scan	This special ultrasound scan measures the thickness of the fold of skin and fluid at the back of the baby's neck. It is usually performed at 11–14 weeks of pregnancy; abnormal thickness may indicate chromosome problems such as Down's syndrome.
Papanicolaou test (smear)	A smear test is used to detect uterine and cervical cancer: a wooden spatula is passed through the cervix to scrape off surface cells, which are transferred onto a glass slide and examined microscopically (not routine but may be offered at your antenatal booking or at your post-natal follow-up appointment).
triple test	A blood test which is offered between 15–20 weeks of pregnancy to test for Down's syndrome.

(Contd)

Test	Reason for test
ultrasound scan	This technique visualizes internal body structure by recording reflections (echoes) of ultrasonic waves. It is used to confirm the stage of pregnancy, postion of the placenta, to estimate the size of the baby and amount of fluid, to identify abnormalities in the baby or diagnose twins.

CASE STUDY

'There's a history of Down's syndrome in my family and because I'm quite late having my first baby we decided to have the amniocentesis test to check she was OK. It was frightening having the test done but the worst bit was waiting for the results – every day I convinced myself there'd be something wrong, but in the end the results were fine.'

Fay, 39, expecting her first baby with partner Laurie, 38

Beauty tips for self-confidence during pregnancy

After the first trimester, many of the early symptoms will diminish or disappear completely and you will probably feel at your most comfortable in the middle three months of pregnancy. Although not every woman feels 'blooming', you may feel better than you have for some time and start to look forward to having your baby and becoming a mother. Unless you are really unwell, use this as a positive excuse to enjoy some of the attention you will no doubt receive, to spend some time (and money if you can spare it) on yourself and to explore ways of harnessing the inner beauty that comes with being pregnant. Use your pregnancy as a time to experiment with new looks for your face, hair and body but also to appreciate how your beauty is quite naturally enhanced, simply by being pregnant.

FACE

▶ *An increased blood supply causes your facial skin to look 'blooming' and you may need to use less foundation make-up than normal.*

▶ *Avoid make-up containing retinoids which reduce wrinkles but contain vitamin A, toners containing salicylic acid, and soy-based lotions and creams, especially if you have very dark pigmentation areas such as the 'mask of pregnancy' (a temporary discolouration of the face, mainly around the cheeks, caused by the pregnancy hormones) or chloasma (unless the products contain 'active soy' in which the soy has been removed).*

▶ *Dry skin usually becomes beautifully supple, giving you a wonderful complexion but oily skin may lead to facial spots as hormone levels increase – ensure your face is kept scrupulously clean and always remove make-up before going to bed.*

▶ *If you develop acne, wash your face twice daily with water and pat dry, use only oil-free make-up products and resist the temptation to squeeze spots. A facial spray containing tea-tree essential oil can reduce spots and help to prevent infection spreading (avoid getting it in your eyes; wash out immediately with cold running water if this happens).*

▶ *Small thin spider veins around your nose and mouth, due to increased blood supply and hormonal effects on blood vessel walls, can develop and are usually permanent. Eat foods rich in vitamin C and use a face cream containing vitamin E.*

HAIR

▶ *Hair grows quickly and may become thicker during pregnancy and much less will fall out, although it does tend to come out in handfuls after you have had your baby. Unfortunately, hair elsewhere can also grow more quickly, including underarm, pubic and leg hair.*

▶ *Hair removal creams and depilatory agents should be used with caution as skin is more sensitive: read the manufacturer's* information carefully and do not use on broken skin. It may be sensible to test a tiny amount on a small area of skin and leave it for 24 hours to see if you develop a reaction, before using the cream on larger areas.

▶ Professional waxing appears to be safe although skin may be more sensitive than normal. Electrolysis is best avoided and may be unnecessary since excess hair falls out after delivery.

▶ Sometimes hair can appear to fall out in pregnancy, but it is likely to be dry hair becoming drier, damaged and brittle, then breaking near the roots. Avoid brushing hair too vigorously and use a mild shampoo and conditioner.

▶ There is divided opinion among doctors about the safety of hair colouring agents in pregnancy; refrain until at least 14 weeks and if possible use chemical-free (organic) substances or go for highlights so less of the colouring agent is absorbed into your body. If you use home colouring kits be warned that your hair may react differently – the colour may 'take' quicker, so rinse off sooner than when not pregnant.

▶ Having a perm or hair straightening is not advisable as hormones affect chemicals used in the products, so either the treatment will not work at all or you will have an over-reaction and hair may be badly damaged.

SKIN

▶ Skin stretches as you gain weight, often leading to stretch marks, which are unfortunately permanent, although they do fade after pregnancy. There is very little you can do to prevent them as proprietary creams cannot penetrate to underlying skin tissues, but weight control may help. Eat fresh foods containing plenty of vitamins and drink as much water as you can to keep skin hydrated.

▶ Increase in pigmentation is due to melanin, influenced by the hormone, oestrogen, so Caucasian women may tan well in the sun without really trying – but do wear sun block and take care not to burn. The use of sunbeds is not recommended – there is some preliminary evidence that excessive UV exposure *may lead to folic acid deficiency, which can adversely affect your pregnancy and your baby.*

▶ *Fake tanning products are relatively safe in pregnancy but allergic reactions are more common as skin is more sensitive; you will still need to use sun block to protect your skin from burning.*

▶ *Moles and freckles will also become darker, but inform your doctor if moles start to bleed, become red, tender or change shape and size.*

▶ *Skin can become sensitive – change to hypoallergenic beauty products.*

▶ *Cellulite can get worse in pregnancy but usually improves again after delivery, especially if you breastfeed your baby.*

▶ *Occasionally little skin tags can develop where skin rubs under clothes, e.g. under your bra line, due to rapid skin growth caused by pregnancy hormones. They are harmless and usually disappear after delivery. It is best to avoid under-wired bras, which put pressure on the developing milk duct system.*

FEET AND HANDS

▶ *Fingernails grow more quickly in mid-pregnancy but also become more brittle or softer. A regular manicure may help – or use lashings of hand and cuticle repair cream.*

▶ *It is probably safe to have acrylic nails applied during pregnancy. However, take care if you are a beautician working in constant proximity to both the chemicals and the vapours from them.*

▶ *Many pregnant women develop a line of very hard skin around the outer edge of the heel as pregnancy progresses, probably due to changes in the centre of gravity that occurs as your 'bump' grows and you tilt backwards. Use lots of moisturizing creams, ask your partner to give you a foot massage, soak your feet regularly in water with foot spa products or essential oils, or treat yourself to a pedicure.*

▶ *Feet grow and widen slightly, due to weight gain and oedema (swelling). This causes shoes to stretch, especially leather ones, so do not wear too many different pairs towards the end of*

*pregnancy as they may be too big afterwards and you will be
unable to wear them.*

▶ *You may also need to think about shoes if you normally wear
high heels, as they may no longer be comfortable and you are
at increased risk of stumbling when pregnant, which can lead
to injury such as a twisted ankle.*

Coping with physical discomforts

Unfortunately, pregnancy tends to take over and control your body
and there is not much that you can do about it except to try and
cope with all the changes. If you fight against what is happening it
will be more difficult to come to terms with it, so try to maintain
a positive attitude to everything and tell yourself that it will all
be worth it in the end. The following section looks at some of the
common discomforts that many expectant mothers experience
and gives suggestions for how you can help yourself to feel better.
Where complementary therapies have been suggested you should
also refer to Part four on Using complementary therapies safely in
pregnancy and childbirth.

'MORNING SICKNESS'

Sickness affects up to 90 per cent of pregnant women and may
occur any time of the day or night, not just in the morning. It
may also last much longer than the first three months, which is
what most of the books for mothers (and professional textbooks
for midwives and doctors) will tell you. It is worse if you are
tired, hungry, anxious, expecting twins, or if you are prone to
travel sickness, and may be accompanied by heartburn, food
cravings or aversions, excessive saliva or headaches. Pregnancy
sickness is mainly due to hormones, but it is also thought to be a
protective mechanism for your baby by preventing you from eating
potentially harmful foods. There may, in some cases, be a link
with thyroid problems, digestive infection or disturbance in the
production of serotonin, one of the brain's 'feel good' chemicals.

Top tip

Hang on to the thought that nausea and vomiting is normal, as it means that the hormone levels are high enough to maintain your pregnancy and provide protection for your baby, allowing him to grow and develop normally.

Self-help and natural therapies for 'morning sickness'

Strategy	How to use it
Nutrition	• Experiment and eat only foods that make you feel better. • Do not feel guilty about not eating a nourishing diet at present. • Do not allow yourself to become too hungry as low blood sugar makes the nausea worse. • Eat carbohydrate for energy but avoid fried or spicy foods.
Herbal remedies *Ginger is not suitable or safe for everyone, peppermint maybe a good alternative.*	• *Avoid* ginger biscuits that have too little ginger and too much sugar to be effective and can make symptoms worse. • Maximum amount: 1 gm of grated raw ginger per day as a tea. • *Do not* take ginger for more than three weeks as it may thin your blood and increase the risk of bleeding – avoid ginger completely if you are taking blood thinning (anticoagulant) drugs, aspirin or tablets for high blood pressure. • Peppermint tea eases heartburn; chewing gum may reduce excess saliva. • Avoid peppermint if you have epilepsy, a heart condition, or a family history of the rare hereditary disorder G6PD. Also avoid if you are taking homeopathic remedies as it stops them from working properly.

(Contd)

Strategy	How to use it
Acupuncture/ acupuncture	• Acupressure wristbands, usually used for travel sickness, are cheap and effective (see Figure 5.1). • Visit an acupuncturist for more individualized treatment.
Homeopathy *Select the remedy most appropriate to your; individual symptoms.* See also Part four.	• *Nux vomica*: nausea is worst in morning; you feel ravenous; crave coffee, tea, alcohol; have constipation with backache, and are usually a 'workaholic'. • *Ipecacuanha*: nausea is constant, especially in the morning; you vomit frequently crave cold drinks; suffer heartburn and headaches; feel anxious and irritable. • *Sepia*: nausea is worst in morning and evening but intermittent all day; worse when hungry; you crave sour foods; want to be alone; are dark and tall in appearance. • *Pulsatilla*: nausea persists all day and is worst late afternoon and evening; you forget to drink; have heartburn and wind; are fair-haired and feminine in appearance; tearful but changeable. • *Cocculus*: best remedy for motion sickness. • *Colchicum*: best remedy for sickness made worse by odours.
Relaxation	• Get plenty of rest and consider time off work. • Try tai ch'i, yoga, listening to music and visualization. • Hypnotherapy/hypnosis CDs can ease stress and anxiety that may make sickness worse.
Other therapies	• Try Morningwell™ CD if sickness is made worse by movement – there is a link between the balancing mechanism in your ear and the vomiting centre in your brain (see Taking it further). • See an osteopath or chiropractor if you have a back or neck problem, which can increase the severity of pregnancy sickness.

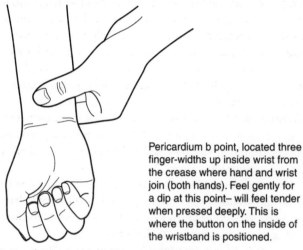

Pericardium b point, located three finger-widths up inside wrist from the crease where hand and wrist join (both hands). Feel gently for a dip at this point– will feel tender when pressed deeply. This is where the button on the inside of the wristband is positioned.

Figure 5.1 Position of acupressure wrist bands to ease 'morning sickness'.

BACKACHE, SCIATICA AND SYMPHYSIS PUBIS PAIN

Backache is very common in pregnancy; as the hormones relax joints, ligaments and muscles, and weight gain increases the curve in the small of your back. Pain can occur in your lower back, shoulders or neck; increasing breast size can cause rib and breastbone discomfort, and may trigger heartburn. Sciatica, an intermittent sharp shooting pain down your legs, is caused by compression of the sciatic nerve. Pubic or pelvic girdle pain (formerly called symphysis pubis discomfort or SPD) occurs because hormones cause instability in the front of your pelvis. Walking, prolonged sitting or standing in one position make it worse. Pain in the coccyx (tailbone), caused by tiny fractures resulting from a fall or previous difficult delivery can flare up in pregnancy – the only treatment is rest.

Stand up straight and tall, pointing your chin downwards to prevent your head tilting backwards. As you become more heavily pregnant there is a tendency to tilt backwards to compensate for your increasing weight and the 'bump' in front: tuck your bottom and coccyx (tailbone) inwards by tilting your pelvis. In bed, use pillows for support; keep your thighs parallel to prevent your top leg twisting across your body (recovery position). When getting out of bed or up from the examination couch in the antenatal clinic, roll onto one side to avoid stretching ligaments, push yourself up to a sitting position, then slowly stand up. When walking, do not force yourself to keep going if you feel uncomfortable, as you risk straining pelvic and back ligaments. If you have very young children, ask them to climb up to you rather than bending down to lift them – and *never* carry a toddler on one hip because this puts great strain on one side of your body. Use a trolley when shopping and carry small bags in both hands rather than a single large one. Where possible, consider shopping online for large or heavy items. Ask the family to help with housework and chores or if you can afford it, pay someone to come in once a week to do heavier tasks such as vacuuming. If possible, sit down to iron or press just a few items at a time. Ask someone to empty the dishwasher to avoid constant bending and to clean round the bath and vacuum the floor so you do not have to stretch. Wear comfortable shoes with broad supporting heels and avoid strappy sandals except for special occasions. Get professionally fitted for a maternity bra so your breasts are properly supported by wide straps and adequately sized cups. A properly fitted bra avoids extra strain on your shoulders and rib cage, which can cause more pain between your shoulders and in your neck. Many high street stores offer a bra fitting service free of charge.

When driving, sit tall, make yourself comfortable so that your back and neck are not stretched or twisted – and *then* adjust your rear view mirror. You may need to adjust the mirror each morning and evening as your posture changes during the day due to gravitational effects. At work, use extra cushions for support or ask for an orthopaedic chair; keep both feet on the floor and do not cross your legs. Leave your desk regularly to move about, preferably at least once an hour. Readjust your computer screen so that you are not hunched over the keyboard and place your mouse mat close enough to avoid stretching. If your work involves standing, try shifting from one foot to the other to ease aches, and sit down when you can.

Natural techniques for backache, sciatica and pubic discomfort

Strategy	How to use it
Massage and aromatherapy *Massage yourself, ask your partner to do it or consult a therapist.* See also Part four.	• Avoid direct thumb or finger pressure in the small of your back where there are acupuncture points, which can stimulate labour. • Shoulder, neck and head massage is good. Avoid deep kneading above your collar bone as there are more acupuncture points here. • Avoid direct massage over areas of sciatica (shooting pain down your legs) until the true cause is known. • Add ylang ylang or lavender oils to your bath – up to four drops in a teaspoon of base oil – these are relaxing and pain relieving.

(Contd)

Strategy	How to use it
Specific postural therapies	• Osteopathy and chiropractic are particularly effective. • Try reflexology, craniosacral therapy or acupuncture. • A physiotherapist will show you special exercises to practise.
Other self-help strategies	• Wear a maternity belt or girdle to support your back. • Paracetamol, 1–2 tablets at four-hourly intervals, can be taken occasionally, but do not to exceed the specified dose. • See your doctor if you are in severe or constant pain, or have other symptoms, e.g. constipation, urinary discomfort, bleeding or abdominal pain.
Homeopathy *Select the remedy most appropriate to your individual symptoms.* See also Part four.	• *Nux vomica*: aching, bruised, dragging ache in lower back; urge to defecate but with constipation; worse in morning and in bed. • *Phosphorus*: pain in lower back and between shoulders; better if massaged; sensitive to cold; you need sympathy. • *Sepia*: pain in small of back; worse in afternoon and at night or when bending or sitting; better if walking; you feel 'worn out' and exhausted; sensitive to cold.

Constipation

Constipation is a reduction in your normal bowel frequency, and is common in pregnancy because the hormone, progesterone, relaxes and slows down peristalsis – intestinal (gut) movement. If you are prone to constipation, it is likely to be worse when you are pregnant, also if you are vomiting frequently or not drinking enough fluid. Some iron tablets given to treat anaemia can add to constipation, although these are not given routinely nowadays: if you do need an iron supplement, try a herbal multivitamin preparation such as Floradix™, eat extra red meat and dark green vegetables, or ask your doctor to change you to a different brand of iron tablet. Always take your iron tablets with orange juice to aid absorption. It is important to prevent constipation or to treat it early, not because it leads to any medical complications but because it is uncomfortable and can make haemorrhoids (piles) prolapse outwards. Avoid eating bran and bran foods unless you at least double your intake of fluid, because it will simply cause more blockage and may interfere with your body's ability to absorb vitamins and minerals from your food. If constipation becomes a more serious problem, your midwife or doctor may prescribe a laxative – these are safe to use in pregnancy but can be rather purgative.

Coping with constipation

Strategy	How to use it
Diet	• Drink three litres of water daily and reduce tea consumption. • Start the day with boiled water with lemon slices. • Begin meals with high fibre raw food – salad, vegetables, fruit. • High fibre foods include oranges, grapefruits, tangerines, blackcurrants, dried prunes and apricots, celery, cherries, watercress, cabbage, spinach and artichokes.
Toilet habits	• While sitting on the lavatory, breathe deeply then exhale, allowing your pelvic floor muscles to relax, but try not to strain. • Ensure time and privacy to go to the toilet. • Stand up to pass the stool – have one knee bent and put your foot on a stool or the edge of the bath.

(Contd)

Strategy	How to use it
Natural remedies	• Try dandelion or mallow leaf tea, steeped in boiling water, drunk daily. • Add three or four drops of orange aromatherapy oil to a teaspoonful of carrier oil and put this in your bath. • Try psyllium husks – but avoid if you have any heart problems.
Manual techniques	• Reflexology – massage the arches of your feet in a clockwise movement to stimulate gut movement. • Massage your abdomen if comfortable. • Acupressure – press intermittently 20–30 times on an acupuncture point in the middle of your abdomen, about three finger widths below your navel. • Consult a registered osteopath or chiropractor.
Homeopathy *Select the remedy most appropriate to your individual symptoms.* See also Part four.	• *Nux vomica*: large hard stools; backache; worse if you drink water; you are irritable, quarrelsome and a 'workaholic'. • *Sepia*: large hard stools; bloating; worse at lunchtime and in evening; better if you exercise; you are indifferent, snappy and weary. • *Pulsatilla*: watery, slimy, greenish-yellow stools; indigestion; worse if you are hot and at night; better if you eat and are in fresh air; you have changeable moods and are emotional. • *Lycopodium*: hard knotty stools; wind; have a feeling of being 'unfinished'; worse if you are hot and between 4 and 8 p.m.; better with warm drink; you are anxious, lack self-confidence but put on a 'brave face'. • *Phosphorus*: long, thin, tough stools passed with difficulty; feel debilitated but have no pain; have ice-cold hands and feet; feel better in the mornings; need sympathy.

HAEMORRHOIDS (PILES)

Haemorrhoids are varicose veins in the rectum and anus, caused by hormones which relax all the veins in the body and commonly develop towards the end of pregnancy when the weight of your baby adds a downwards pressure to your pelvic floor, sometimes causing the haemorrhoids to protrude outwards (prolapse). They are likely to occur earlier or be worse if you have gained a lot of extra weight, are expecting more than one baby or have had them before. They can feel itchy or painful after having your bowels open and may bleed. It is important to check that any bleeding is from your haemorrhoids, not from your uterus – if you are unsure ask your midwife for advice. Conventional treatment usually involves prescribing creams or lotions to apply to the outside of the piles – a local anaesthetic gel to put around the outer rim of the anus just before you attempt to have your bowels open may help to reduce the additional pain you can sometimes feel with the downwards pressure of the stool.

Dealing with haemorrhoids

Strategy	How to use it
Diet	• Avoid constipation – see above. • Reduce refined carbohydrates, e.g. sweets, white bread and white rice. • Avoid bran unless you double your fluid intake.
Natural remedies and other therapies	• Apply hammamelis/witch hazel directly to visible piles to shrink them. • Try cypress or frankincense aromatherapy oils in the bath, four drops. • Rescue Remedy cream, applied directly can ease discomfort. • Consult an acupuncturist, reflexologist or osteopath.

(Contd)

Strategy	How to use it

Homeopathy
Select the remedy most appropriae to your individual symptoms.
See also Part four.

- *Pulsatilla*: you have large, congested bleeding piles that itch; you feel emotional and tearful; need reassurance; you may also have varicose veins and/or heartburn and indigestion.
- *Nux vomica*: you have grape-like, congested piles; burning; constipation with backache; feel worse at night; better if you bathe in cold water; are irritable, sensitive and quarrelsome.
- *Sepia*: you have congested painful, bleeding piles that protrude when straining and feel like a hard mass in rectum; are sensitive to cold but perspire easily; exhausted, worn out, do not want sympathy.
- *Lycopodium*: you have large, chronic, blue-purplish bleeding, itching piles which protrude during defecation; constipation; you crave sweet things; lack self-confidence but put on a 'brave face'.

HEARTBURN AND INDIGESTION

Heartburn, indigestion and acid regurgitation usually occur in late pregnancy due to the progesterone which relaxes the valve at the entrance to your stomach, causing a small amount of acid to surge upwards into your oesophagus (gullet), triggering burning pain in the middle of your chest. Sometimes heartburn accompanies 'morning sickness' in earlier pregnancy. If your baby is big or in the breech position (bottom first) or if you are expecting twins, these symptoms will be more severe due to pressure under your diaphragm; certain foods and smoking may also exacerbate them. Your midwife or doctor may suggest antacid medicine but many women dislike the taste; also, excessive use may interfere with your body's ability to absorb other minerals from your food – this is especially relevant to preparations containing aluminium.

Self-help for heartburn

Therapy	How to use it
Self-help methods	• Use several pillows at night to prevent pressure on the stomach valve. • Take a *maximum of one-quarter teaspoon* of sodium bicarbonate (baking soda) in water between meals to neutralize stomach acid.
Diet	• Avoid foods which aggravate symptoms – rich, spicy, fried, greasy foods, tea, coffee, alcohol, sugar and E additives in processed foods. • Eat small frequent meals to avoid pressure on the valve from an overfull stomach. • Eat raw garlic daily or take a good quality garlic capsule rich in allicin, the active ingredient, to reduce symptoms.
Natural remedies	• Try ginger, camomile or dandelion root tea or slippery elm tablets (avoid dandelion if you are diabetic as it may affect blood sugar levels, or if you are on drugs for high blood pressure). • Try four drops of lemon, orange or neroli aromatherapy oils with one drop of black pepper essential oil in 5 ml of base oil to massage your chest and upper back.
Other therapies	• Complementary therapies to correct or adapt your posture may be helpful, including yoga, t'ai chi or the Alexander technique.

(Contd)

Therapy	How to use it

Homeopathy
Select the remedy most appropriate to your individual symptoms.
See also Part four.

- **Nux vomica**: you have bitter, sour reflux; a metallic taste; feel bloated and heavy; experience cramping stomach pain; are worse after eating and when wearing tight clothing; better with hot drinks; are irritable, sensitive and quarrelsome.
- **Pulsatilla**: you have bitter, sour reflux, which tastes of food just eaten; leaves slimy or salty taste; have an empty feeling in stomach; feel worse in evening and after rich, fatty food, bread, milk, fruit or meat; are emotional and tearful; need sympathy.
- **Natrum mur**: you have watery, sweet reflux; abdominal cramps; feel worse if you eat starchy food; better if you do not eat; keep emotions to yourself; cry when alone.
- **Causticum**: you have fatty, greasy reflux; stomach feels full, are worse when walking, wet or cold and in evening; better if you are warm or have hot drinks; you cry a lot and despair of feeling better.

Insight

Although the herbal remedy, ginger, can ease mild heartburn in some women, too much can actually cause heartburn and indigestion, so if you are have 'morning sickness' with heartburn, don't take ginger which will make it worse.

HEADACHES

Headaches are fairly normal in early pregnancy. They are usually triggered by the relaxing effects of progesterone on the blood vessels in the brain and head. Tiredness, anxiety and stress, 'morning sickness' or eyesight problems, noise, dehydration and travelling to and from work may make them more severe.

Migraines can also worsen in early pregnancy but usually settle down later. However, in later pregnancy, headaches may be a symptom of pre-eclampsia (pregnancy high blood pressure). Always tell your midwife if you have unexpected headaches after 24 weeks of pregnancy, especially if they are focused around the front of your head and over your eyes.

It is acceptable very occasionally to take small doses of painkillers such as paracetamol but do not take more than the recommended dose; ibuprofen and aspirin are best avoided completely unless prescribed by your doctor. Discontinue the paracetamol if they have no real effect and speak to your midwife or doctor for advice. It may also be worth consulting an optician to check your eyesight, as pregnancy oedema (fluid retention) can affect the shape and size of the eyeball – if you wear contact lenses this can also cause friction and irritation on the eye surface and you may need spectacles during pregnancy instead of your lenses. Avoid eating stimulating foods, e.g. chocolate, cheese, coffee, tea, alcohol, cola and processed foods containing additives and preservatives and drink plenty of water. Eat regularly to maintain your blood sugar levels. Other simple things that may help include resting in a cool darkened room, having a warm (not hot) bath, or getting some fresh air and gentle exercise. Yoga, t'ai chi, swimming or relaxation techniques such as deep breathing may also help. Try gentle neck and head exercises – slowly rotate your head to one side as far as you can, return to the mid-line and repeat in the opposite direction. Lift your shoulders and then allow them to drop downwards as far as possible from your ears; slowly lift and stretch one arm, circle forwards then backwards, lower and repeat with the other arm.

Insight

Headaches in late pregnancy, especially around the front of your head 'like a vice', may be associated with high blood pressure and worsening pre-eclampsia, because swelling, from fluid retention, develops around your brain and eyes, in the same way as you can develop swollen ankles.

Relieving headaches

Strategy	How to use it
Natural remedies See also Part four	• Use lavender and/or peppermint essential oil, one drop of each neat, rubbed gently into your temples or drink lavender or peppermint tea. • Bach flower remedies may help, e.g. olive if you are tired, impatiens if you are irritable or Rescue Remedy if you are stressed. • Tiger balm is a popular headache remedy but its safety in pregnancy is not known, as it contains camphor, so is probably best avoided.
Manual therapies	• Massage your temples or your whole head in a 'hair washing' movement, or treat yourself to an Indian head massage. • A simple home reflexology treatment is to massage your own big toes gently as they correspond to the zone for the head and neck. • Osteopathy, chiropractic and acupuncture are all effective in treating headaches, especially if you also have related back problems.
Homeopathy *Select the remedy most appropriate to your individual symptoms.* See also Part four.	• *Sepia*: you have throbbing shooting pain over your left eye which is worse when travelling or if you bend; better after eating and in fresh air; you feel ambivalent, intolerant and confused. • *Chamomilla*: you have a pulsating, tearing pain; feel worse if you drink coffee or eat sweets; better after eating and changing position; feel irrationally angry. • *Belladonna*: you have a pounding headache; worse with jarring movement, especially in the afternoon; better in morning; are nervous, restless, fearful; may be pregnant during the summer months. • *Aconite*: you have a throbbing, bursting headache which develops suddenly; feel worse if cold; better when resting and in open air; are irritable and very sensitive to pain.

CARPAL TUNNEL SYNDROME

Tingling and pain in your wrists can result from fluid retention, which compresses the channel of nerves (the carpal tunnel), which runs up your arm. You may lose manual dexterity and coordination, finding it difficult to make fine movements with your fingers and thumb and to grip things. It can be particularly painful in the morning as your hands curl up while you are asleep – your midwife may provide you with hand splints to wear at night to reduce this, although they are not particularly comfortable to wear. Carpal tunnel syndrome usually occurs towards the end of pregnancy and is likely to recur in a subsequent pregnancy. It usually disappears after the birth when hormone and fluid levels return to normal, although it can persist for some weeks, sometimes worsening in the first few days after delivery in the same way as swollen ankles. If the problem continues after you have had your six-week post-natal examination, consult your doctor who may refer you for a specialist medical opinion; prolonged carpal tunnel syndrome may need to be treated with surgery.

Easing carpal tunnel syndrome

Strategy	How to use it
Self-help methods	• Try 'wrist wringing'– clasp one wrist with your other hand, massage in a circular movement ('Chinese burn'), repeat on the other hand. • Avoid painful movements; exercise your hands and arms gently to stretch them. • Hang your hands over the sides of the bed at night. • Try putting your hands in cold water for a while.

(Contd)

Strategy	How to use it

Aromatherapy and herbal remedies. See also Part four

- Try a compress of cypress and chamomile essential oils – soak a cloth in warm or cool water to which four drops have been added and wrap it around your wrists.
- Drinking chamomile tea may reduce inflammation.
- Wrap dark green cabbage leaves, cooled in the refrigerator, around your wrists (wipe but do not wash). Leave until they become wet. Repeat until your wrists feels better – osmotic pressure draws out excess fluid. This is also good for swollen ankles.
- *Avoid* juniper berry oil (quoted in some books as good for swelling), especially if you have kidney disease or diabetes.

Manual techniques

- Try reflexology 'first aid': imagine a line on the upper surface of each foot below the fourth toe – about 2 cm up from the nail you will find a tender spot – press firmly with your thumb, until the tenderness goes. Repeat four or five times until no longer painful (see Figure 5.2).

Homeopathy *Select the remedy most appropriate to your individual Symptoms.* See also Part four.

- *Apis*: you have tingling and numbness radiating up your left arm; swollen wrists and first and second fingers; you feel better if you move your wrist, worse when hot; are tearful, irritable, restless, jealous.
- *Causticum*: you have tingling and numbness in fingers but no swelling; pain is worse in fingertips and thumb, especially in the morning; you are anxious, sensitive, pessimistic, sensitive to cold.
- *Lycopodium*: you have tingling and numbness in all fingers except little (fifth) finger, with some wrist swelling; feel worse at night and on waking; are restless, anxious and fearful but put on a 'good face'.
- *Calcarea carb*: you have tingling, numbness and swelling in wrists and first three fingers; are anxious, sluggish, have poor concentration; feel cold but perspire profusely.

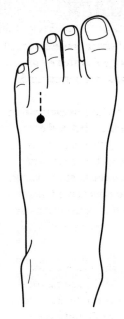

Upper surface of both feet, below fourth toe; about 2 cm locate slight dip. Press this point firmly (will feel tender) until tenderness subsides. Repeat several times until wrist/hand pain eases.

Figure 5.2 Reflexology point to treat carpal tunnel syndrome.

10 THINGS TO REMEMBER

1 *Physical symptoms of pregnancy, such as nausea, backache, varicose veins and constipation are normal – but if they are excessively strong or have prolonged symptoms, check with your midwife.*

2 *Your breasts increase several sizes – make sure you get fitted early for a supportive bra.*

3 *Try to avoid sitting up too quickly when you get up, or lying flat on your back in late pregnancy, as the effects of changes in your circulation mean that your blood pressure fluctuates and can cause you to feel dizzy.*

4 *It is normal to need to pass urine frequently in pregnancy but if you have any burning or discomfort, tell your midwife who can check for infection.*

5 *Eat plenty of fruit, vegetables and fibre foods to keep healthy and drink plenty of fluid to prevent constipation.*

6 *STOP or reduce smoking and alcohol consumption, as well as any other harmful substances you may take.*

7 *If you take medication for a medical condition, you should only change or reduce it after discussing it with your doctor.*

8 *Be aware of the things you are advised to stop eating during pregnancy, but do not become obsessed with doing 'what's right' about everything.*

9 *You will normally have an early antenatal appointment with the midwife who will record your medical history and use it to help plan your pregnancy care, and who*

will arrange for various tests and investigations that may be necessary.

10 *If you are unsure, or worried, always ask your midwife to explain the tests and investigations you are offered: you do have the right to decline them.*

Part one: positive pregnancy – the end of the beginning

Now that you have read this Positive pregnancy section, you will hopefully have given some thought to your own situation and may have worked out a few ways in which you can cope with any difficulties you experience. The one incontrovertible fact is that pregnancy definitely has an end in sight – the birth of your baby – so it cannot last forever. Despite the fact that many millions of women conceive, are pregnant and give birth every day this may be one of the very few times that *you* will do it. Congratulate yourself on your abilities, recognize your strengths and do not feel guilty about your weaknesses. Applaud yourself and your baby for getting to your pregnancy destination – the birth – and get ready to welcome him into the world.

Top tip
Remember: Think positive!

Part two

Positive parturition (childbirth)

6

Emotions and feelings

In this chapter you will learn:
- *how to stay in control by deciding where to give birth*
- *how to prepare for the 'big day'*
- *how to remain assertive by understanding your choices in labour.*

Having a baby is arguably the most significant thing that will ever occur in your life and that of your partner and it is understandable that you will feel a range of emotions, particularly as the date of your baby's birth approaches. You will hopefully, by now, feel excited and keen to meet your baby but you may also be feeling anxious, perhaps even a little afraid of what is to come, which is partly, of course, due to fear of the unknown. No one knows what will happen during labour because it is so unpredictable – even if you have had several other children, every labour is different. You will probably be intrigued about what the experience will be like and may be wondering if you will be able to cope with labour contractions – especially if friends and relatives have told you 'horror' stories about their own experiences. You will obviously also be concerned for your baby – despite anything that may happen during the labour you will want him/her to be born alive and well. Remember, however, that childbirth is a natural, normal life event and will, in the majority of women, proceed without any problems. Statistically, you have about a 70 per cent chance of having your baby normally without any complications. If you are basically fit and healthy and your pregnancy has progressed well, it is highly likely that your labour will proceed normally – and if you do have any specific medical or pregnancy problems, you will obviously want to have the best care available to ensure that your baby is all right.

It is important to prepare yourself for the birth, but you will be pleased to know that nature takes a hand to make the 'run up' to the 'big day' a little easier. As labour gets closer, pregnancy hormone levels, which have prevented your uterus from contracting, start to decrease, allowing labour hormones to be produced. This makes your Braxton Hicks contractions (painless pregnancy contractions which aid flow of oxygen to your baby) stronger as your uterus becomes 'irritable' in readiness for labour. At the same time your body's stress hormone levels change and the 'feel good' chemicals increase, making you feel mentally more prepared for the impending birth and better able to cope with it. This seems to be nature's way of helping us towards labour. It is probable, in any case, that you will, by now, be so fed up with being pregnant and so desperate to meet your baby face-to-face that labour and the birth eventually become a welcome release from the discomforts and uncertainties of pregnancy. Additionally, although many mothers worry about coping with labour, contractions should never be worse than your body can cope with. If you do find it difficult to cope, there are several ways in which your midwife or therapist can help you to feel more comfortable – see Working with contractions in Chapter 9.

Insight

Your uterine muscle is like a piece of elastic, tight and difficult to stretch at first, which is why first labours are normally the longest. Second and third labours are normally quicker because the 'elastic' muscles have already been stretched once. However, by the time you get to your fourth or fifth labour, this 'elastic' is tired and overstretched and needs to work harder to do the same amount of work as before: this is why, if you have more than four babies, the labours are likely to be longer and perhaps more difficult.

If this is not your first baby, it is also natural for you to think about previous birth experiences, both good, and perhaps not so good. First labours are usually the longest, but every labour and birth is different. If you had complications in a previous labour, you may be wondering whether they will occur again, for example if you will need another Caesarean section or forceps delivery. Talk to your midwife or obstetrician and ask as many questions as possible to help set your mind at rest. If you are particularly concerned, it can be useful to seek professional help to 'de-brief' about your previous experiences before you go into labour this time (see Taking it further).

Insight

Childbirth is the most fundamental human activity, which aims to continue the human race.

In the vast majority of women it is normal – it is what your body is designed to do.

Childbirth is an emotionally charged event, which evokes many differing feelings in each of the people present at the birth, some of which are instantaneous and short-lived while others will bring lifelong memories. Some people may experience emotions based on their own previous life experiences, and sometimes feelings become so overwhelming that they elicit physical manifestations, causing completely unexpected reactions. It is certainly not unusual for those present at the birth of a baby to shed a tear or feel choked by emotion. Conversely, the intensity of the event and the anxiety experienced by many onlookers, particularly the partner, can cause some to display uncharacteristically negative emotions such as anger, irritability or rudeness. This is normal and not unexpected (even if it can occasionally make things difficult).

Where to give birth to your baby

Remember that this is your baby and you are entitled to choose where to have him, according to your wishes and personal and family circumstances. Making informed decisions can help you to remain in control. You can plan to deliver your baby at home, in a birth centre or in a maternity unit at your local hospital but be prepared to be flexible as things can change throughout your pregnancy, which may mean that your planned place of birth needs to change. You may be given a formal choice by your maternity professionals, although many doctors try to discourage you from having a home birth. In order to make your decision, think about whether this is your first baby and if not, how you coped with any previous labours, whether you are expecting more than one baby or whether you or your baby have any particular medical problems. If you have an existing medical condition, you may be advised to have your baby in hospital as you may be more likely to develop complications. If your baby is very big, very small or premature, it would also be wise to have ready access to more medical facilities than would be available at home. If you are over the age of 40, your doctor may try to persuade you to deliver in hospital as there is a slightly increased risk of complications in older women, although age is not, in itself, a reason for insisting on a hospital birth. Your choice may also depend on where you live and the circumstances of your domestic situation. If you live within easy reach of emergency services, choosing a home birth will not normally be a problem, but if you live in the middle of nowhere down a tiny road which is difficult to negotiate, or if your home does not have reasonable modern conveniences such as running water and lavatory facilities, this can pose certain difficulties at the time of your baby's birth, although these are not insurmountable – and the choice remains yours. The following pages explain some of the advantages and disadvantages of each place of birth.

Insight

The UK government has committed to providing for every mother to give birth at home, if she so wishes, by 2012. However, this is already your choice – you are legally entitled to have your baby wherever you choose, so do not be put off if your doctor tries to tell you otherwise.

HOME BIRTH

Advantages

▶ *Research shows home birth is safe for low-risk women with a midwife present to support them.*
▶ *There is less risk of infection.*
▶ *Labour is more likely to progress normally, without unnecessary interventions.*
▶ *You have privacy, comfort and can have friends and family with you.*
▶ *You are in control.*
▶ *You will have continued attendance of known midwives who will be aware of your particular desires for, and anxieties about, labour.*
▶ *Studies suggest home birth is more cost effective for the State – care is provided only for the time that you need it.*

Disadvantages

▶ *You may have to deal with negative comments from medical staff and others about having your baby at home.*
▶ *It is not possible to have medical interventions in labour such as epidural for pain relief, Caesarean section, forceps delivery, etc.*
▶ *You have more responsibilities, both for your labour care and for ongoing domestic issues, e.g. meals, child care, etc.*
▶ *Your midwife may not reach you in time for the birth so be prepared for this.*
▶ *You may have increased expense, e.g. independent midwife – a home birth is not paid for by medical insurance.*

BIRTH CENTRE

Advantages

▶ *This is a compromise between home and hospital birth.*
▶ *You have greater control and it is similar to being in your own home.*
▶ *You meet the staff before labour, so are normally cared for by a known midwife.*

Disadvantages

▶ *There are strict criteria for accessibility – you may be excluded due to, for example, your age or having rhesus negative blood.*

▶ *You are away from home and family; you need to travel to the centre when in labour.*

▶ *There are no doctors available – if complications arise you would be moved to the main maternity unit for delivery.*

HOSPITAL BIRTH

Advantages

▶ *This is the safest environment for mothers and/or babies at risk of complications.*

▶ *Emergencies can be dealt with promptly; essential equipment is available.*

▶ *This is the only option if Caesarean is necessary.*

▶ *24-hour care – medical, midwifery and other aspects such as meals – is available.*

Disadvantages

▶ *There is a much greater risk of infection.*

▶ *You are more likely to have medical intervention and operative delivery such as Caesarean.*

▶ *The experience is less personal and private, and can be intimidating. There are rules about visitors, etc.*

▶ *You may be left alone for long periods if other mothers have more urgent needs.*

▶ *There is less opportunity to rest after the birth.*

▶ *Your baby may be separated from you for some of the time.*

▶ *You are more likely to receive conflicting advice.*

▶ *It is much more difficult to establish successful breastfeeding.*

'I've chosen to have my baby in the local maternity unit where I know I can have an epidural if I want one and there will be all the facilities if anything goes wrong. Of course, I'm hoping everything will be OK but I just don't want to take the chance.'

Nitisha, 25, expecting her first baby

When you have read this section, you may wish to use the table below to consider each issue in relation to your own circumstances, to help you make a decision about where to have your baby.

MY DECISIONS ABOUT WHERE TO GIVE BIRTH TO MY BABY

Issue	My personal situation and my feelings about it
Safety:	risk of infection; risk of complications in labour; accessibility of emergency services
Interventions:	availability of epidural, induction of labour, Caesarean section, etc.
Companions:	whether it is important to know in advance who will care for you; presence of family, doula, therapist; presence of other children
Medical history:	whether you have any medical or pregnancy conditions; if you have rhesus negative blood; whether a previous labour progressed normally
Attitudes:	whether you feel assertive enough to 'battle' for a home birth; how you feel about staff attitudes and care in local hospital; whether you would prefer to know the doctor/ midwife who provides care
Finances:	whether you can afford to pay for services, e.g. an independent midwife, doula, private obstetrician.

Preparation for labour

Whether you have decided to have your baby at home, in a birth centre, in the maternity unit of your local hospital, or privately, either with a midwife at home or an obstetrician in a private hospital, you will need to organize things for the day of your labour. This helps you to focus your thoughts on the forthcoming birth and to get organized so that you do not feel panicky when you go into labour. Make sure you know how to contact your partner or whoever is going to be with you during labour – it may be a good idea to leave their number near the telephone just in case you forget it in the rush. Some couples who do not have access to a mobile telephone arrange to hire a bleeper for the last few weeks of pregnancy in order to alert the partner when the mother goes into labour. Arrange for someone to look after your other children – even if you are going to be at home it is wise to allocate someone to be on hand to sort out meals, bedtime and keeping them occupied if they do not want to be with you. You may need to ask a neighbour to feed any pets if you are going to hospital, especially if you are having a planned Caesarean and will be away for a few days, or if your partner is going to stay with family or friends.

If you are having your baby at home, your midwife will normally arrange to deliver any necessary equipment a few weeks before your due date, or she may bring it with her on the day. Try to arrange the room in which you intend to labour – clear out unnecessary furniture and perhaps change the room round to ensure as much space as possible. Although you will be encouraged to be up and about during labour, you may want to sit or lie on the bed – if you do not normally sleep in this bed, prepare it beforehand or ask someone to do it for you when you go into labour. After putting on the bottom sheet, place a sheet of thin plastic on top, if possible one that is large enough to tuck in. If you do not have a large enough piece of plastic, cut open plastic bin liners and flatten them out. Over the top of the plastic put another cotton sheet, preferably an old one. Once your baby is born, the top sheet and plastic can be easily removed, and if necessary disposed of, leaving you with a fresh sheet underneath.

Think about what you might like to do, especially during early labour. If you feel you may want to watch television or a film, consider booking a rental DVD or buy one you always wanted to see. If playing games appeals, search out those old board games that never get used or a pack of playing cards. You need games that take a reasonable time to play but do not require too much concentration – word games can be all right in very early labour but may not help later on when you will want to concentrate on coping with your contractions. While you are still in early labour, you could set yourself a task that you have been meaning to do for some time – for example, sorting out all the family photographs into albums, or something else that will not matter if you leave half finished.

If you are planning a home water birth, make sure you have booked the pool and know how to assemble it (they are normally delivered in pieces which slot together). If there is any doubt about the strength of the floor to accommodate a heavy pool of water, check it out before you go into labour. Ensure that the water heater/immersion is turned on so that there will be enough hot water (see also The power of water, in Chapter 9).

Packing for labour

Check you have each of the following:

Items for yourself
- ☐ *Maternity notes and copy of birth plan.*
- ☐ *Clothes for labour: old T-shirt, warm socks, slippers, hairband.*
- ☐ *Clothes for after birth: nightdress or tracksuit, old dark-coloured knickers or paper ones; dressing gown, feeding bra.*
- ☐ *Cosmetic bag: soap, flannel, shampoo, conditioner, toothbrush and toothpaste, face cream; mouthwash, facial refresher spray, lip balm, tissues, deodorant, hairbrush; towels, sanitary pads (not tampons), breast pads.*
- ☐ *Aromatherapy oils, homeopathic and Bach flower remedies, portable fan, oil vaporizer (not electrical if hospital birth); TENS machine, birthing ball, hot water bottle or gel pads.*

- ☐ *Pillow (labelled) or inflatable pillow (hospitals are always short of pillows!); plenty of old towels if you are at home.*
- ☐ *Miscellaneous: pen, birth notification cards, stamps, address book, magazine or book, board games, MP3 or portable CD player and CDs, portable pool.*

Items for partner/baby
- ☐ *Camera or video to record the event.*
- ☐ *Coins for parking and telephone, phone card or mobile phone and relevant numbers.*
- ☐ *Food and drinks – sandwiches, biscuits, water, juice, flask of coffee or money for machine, etc.*
- ☐ *Spare T-shirt, jersey, mouthwash, toothbrush and toothpaste for partner, baby soap, oil, talcum powder, cotton wool balls, towel.*
- ☐ *Baby clothes, vests, all-in-one suits, cardigan, nightgowns, hat, mittens, socks, nappies, plastic pants if needed.*
- ☐ *If you are not breastfeeding your baby you will also need to take formula feed.*
- ☐ *Items for going home: baby car seat, blanket, your own clothes and shoes (often forgotten!).*
- ☐ *Miscellaneous: plastic sheeting to protect bed or car seat.*

Do *not* take large amounts of cash, credit cards or jewellery into hospital/birth centre.

Birth planning

It can be useful to devise a plan for your preferences for labour. Discuss your ideas with your intended birth supporter, then with your midwife so that your choices can be recorded in your maternity notes. Formal birth plans were very much in vogue in the 1980s and 1990s but are not now encouraged routinely, as most midwives believe that care in labour should be individualized to meet your needs and wishes at the time. Birth plans can be rather counter-productive if things do not go according to plan and it is possible that you may be disappointed if you do not achieve everything you had previously decided. You may also change your mind at the last minute, so be prepared to be flexible. However, it is helpful to focus on the different aspects of possible care which you may want or need during labour and the birth of your baby.

You will need to consider various issues, preferably before you go into labour when you may be less able to make objective decisions. For example, you may be advised to have your baby's heart rate monitored continuously throughout labour, but unless there are specific medical reasons, this is not usually essential. Research has shown that continuous unnecessary monitoring can cause more anxiety than being monitored intermittently, especially since professionals tend to focus more on the technology than on you. Other methods of monitoring are available which do not require you to be strapped to a bed or chair, connected to an electronic monitor. There are a few reasons for continuous monitoring, such as premature labour, induction of labour, if you are expecting more than one baby, or if you develop complications, but the choice remains yours. Ask your midwife to explain the reasons if she recommends continuous monitoring, especially if you had decided it is not what you wanted .

How often would you prefer to have internal (vaginal) examinations during labour? An internal examination enables the midwife to determine how far your labour has progressed, dilatation of the cervix, descent of your baby, whether the bag of membranes has broken (and sometimes to break it artificially) and the position of your baby's head. Occasionally, an internal examination is necessary to take blood from the baby's scalp to test his stress levels, as in a very slow or difficult labour. Some midwives believe it is only necessary to perform an internal examination to check your progress when there is an indication to do so, such as before an epidural, whereas others feel it is important to examine you regularly, just in case problems are developing. Talk to your midwife and decide for yourself which option will suit you better, but be guided by your midwife or doctor if labour does not proceed according to plan.

> ### Insight
> An internal (vaginal) examination involves you lying on your back with your legs apart so that the midwife can place her gloved fingers inside your vagina and up to the cervix. In labour this can sometimes be uncomfortable but it usually only takes a few minutes and enables the midwife to 'see' what is happening and how you are progressing.

During the first stage would you like to be able to eat and drink? (Put sandwiches ready in the freezer or stock up on other easily digested carbohydrate snacks you may fancy.) Traditionally, mothers in labour were discouraged from eating as it was thought that, in the event of needing a Caesarean section, there was an increased risk of inhaling acid stomach contents during the anaesthetic. However, contemporary research suggests that it is beneficial to eat carbohydrate snacks to maintain your energy levels. In the event that an emergency Caesarean seems likely, you can be given medicine which neutralizes stomach acid to prevent the problems of inhalation. In any case, the majority of Caesarean sections are now performed under epidural/spinal anaesthetic in which you are wide awake, so the chances of vomiting and inhaling food are very small.

How will you cope with the contractions? Explore the advantages and disadvantages of each method, and perhaps consider some of the complementary therapies and natural remedies available. (See Chapter 9 for more on Working with contractions.) Experiment with different positions during the first stage of labour and think about the position you might like to be in for the actual birth – traditionally women are often propped up on a bed but you could be on 'all fours' or standing or on your side. Have you thought about the possibility of having a water labour – and do you want your baby to be born in the water or would you prefer to get out for the delivery? (See The power of water in Chapter 9.)

Work through your feelings about having an episiotomy (a cut to enlarge the birth opening) at the time of delivery. Although having a surgical cut into your perineum (the area between the lower edge of your vagina and your anus) may sound horrific, some mothers believe it may be better than having a spontaneous tear which can occur if the area is too tight for the baby to come out. However, there is some evidence to suggest that a natural tear will heal better and with less discomfort afterwards (and you do not always need to have stitches), usually because it has only extended in the direction and to the extent needed, whereas an episiotomy is a cut of a specific length in a specific direction. It is advisable to discuss this with your midwife before you go into labour, if possible.

Insight

An episiotomy involves a small anaesthetic injection into the skin between your vaginal opening and your anus; the midwife then uses sterilized scissors to make a single clean cut which enlarges the opening for your baby to be born. Sometimes, if this is not done, the baby struggles to emerge because your perineum is too strong for him and this can lead to distress in your baby, which is why it may be advised by your midwife.

Think about whether or not to have an injection to speed up the third stage of your labour – the delivery of the placenta. It is fairly normal practice for mothers to be offered an artificial hormone to make the uterus contract quickly after the baby's delivery and to control bleeding, but research indicates that, in most mothers, the third stage should proceed normally. Again, you do have the right to refuse, but if you are anaemic or have had bleeding in pregnancy, or if you have specific medical problems such as high blood pressure, you may be actively advised to have the injection. If you are in any doubt about whether or not this is the right decision for you, talk to your midwife in late pregnancy or during early labour.

> If you have anaemia, you have less red blood cells than normal so that any blood loss will have a potentially more serious effect on you than if the same amount were lost if you were not anaemic.

As your baby is being born, do you want to be told the sex or to look and find out for yourself? Do you want your baby to be placed straight up to your breast or would you prefer it if he was dried, washed and wrapped warmly before you hold him? Do you mind if the umbilical cord is cut immediately the baby is born or do you want the midwife to wait until it has stopped pulsating before she cuts it? Does your partner want to cut it – and is this allowed?

What are your feelings about your baby being given vitamin K? Vitamin K helps the blood to clot and although your baby receives some via the placenta, it is not always enough to prevent bleeding, especially in those born prematurely or who have breathing problems, or babies who have had a complicated birth such as a forceps delivery or Caesarean section. A very small number of babies develop bleeding problems for no known reason and it is not really possible to identify those most at risk, so paediatricians believe it is necessary to offer all babies vitamin K after birth. It can be given either as a single injection within a couple of hours of birth, or as three oral doses, although this is less reliable and requires extra appointments with the midwife. Active breastfeeding in the early days can go some way towards preventing the bleeding condition, as the pre-milk, colostrum, contains vitamin K.

Think also about your preferences if you are advised to have an induction of labour or a Caesarean section (see Coping with problems in labour in Chapter 9) or if complications develop. Do you have any other thoughts about this special event in your life? It may take some time to investigate all your options and decide what you want, but when you are ready, you can complete your own plan for the birth, if you wish.

MY PERSONAL PLAN FOR LABOUR AND BIRTH

Decisions I/we have made about the labour and birth of my/our baby	
Preferred place of birth	
Preferred companions during labour and the birth	
Preferences regarding onset of labour/induction	
Things I would like to do to stay comfortable	
Preferred method(s) of pain relief if I need it	
Decisions about the use of complementary therapies/natural remedies	
Preferences for mobility/positions during first stage of labour	
Decision about water labour/birth	
Preferences regarding monitoring of my/our baby's heartbeat	
Preferences regarding eating/drinking in labour	
Preferences regarding internal examinations – routine or as required	
Preferred position for birth of my/our baby	
Preferences regarding episiotomy/tear	
Decision about whether to have baby brought up to breast at birth	
Decision about cutting of the umbilical cord	
Decision about third stage of labour	
Decision about vitamin K for my/our baby	
Decision about method of feeding my/our baby – breast/bottle	
Any other preferences/decisions	

10 THINGS TO REMEMBER

1 *It is natural to be anxious about labour, but as you approach the 'big day' your body will take over: your labour hormones will increase in readiness and this suppresses your stress hormones, so you should feel less anxious the nearer you get.*

2 *Your decision about where to have your baby should be based on a balance between your preferred venue, safety, practical and geographical issues, and the availability of additional services you may require.*

3 *Prepare for labour at least four weeks before your due date – normal labour occurs any time between 37 and 43 weeks of pregnancy.*

4 *If you have particular wishes for your labour you may want to write these on a birth plan, but it is wise to discuss your wishes with your midwife, well in advance of the day.*

5 *You do NOT have to submit to any treatment you do not wish to have, e.g. induction of labour, but always be guided by the advice given by your midwives and doctors and ask for clarification if there is anything you do not fully understand.*

6 *Find out from your midwife about the policies in the unit where you are due to give birth, especially if there are issues that you have particular views on, e.g. induction of labour when overdue.*

7 *If there is anything which you do not wish to have you are at liberty to decline, e.g. continuous monitoring of your baby during labour.*

8 *Make sure you know about the different methods of relieving pain in labour, including steps you can take yourself.*

9   *Talk to your midwife about aspects such as episiotomy,
    vitamin K for your baby, etc.*

10 *If you are having your baby at home, rearrange the
    furniture about four weeks before your due date and make
    arrangements for the midwife to deliver the necessary items
    to you.*

7

....

Sex and relationships

In this chapter you will learn:
- *how to decide who you may want with you during labour*
- *about the professionals involved in maternity care.*

By this time, it is hoped that your partner will be getting as excited as you about the birth of your baby even if he has worries which may be different from your own. For most couples in a loving relationship, pregnancy brings them closer together and can often cause them to reflect on the meaning of life. It can make you feel like an incredibly tiny cog in the vast wheel of the world, or it may reassure you of your significance in continuing the human race. However you feel, it is almost without doubt that your relationship with your partner will change. There may, for example, have been a necessarily practical shift in various activities such as household chores, while stopping work, even temporarily, brings financial challenges for most families. Although sometimes worrying, these factors can contribute to your partner enjoying a greater sense of the traditional role of the man as the 'bread winner' and may make him more protective of you, physically, practically and financially.

As labour approaches, sexual activity may, for some couples, be a dim and distant memory, something that happened before you became tired, heavy and cumbersome. Sexual contact in pregnancy, whether it is full penetrative intercourse or not, can bring new emotional and physical challenges but hopefully also facilitates a renewal or strengthening of your feelings for one another, becoming more loving and creative in late pregnancy (see Chapter 3).

Much has been written about whether birth can be a sexual experience or not, but your thoughts on this may depend on your beliefs about the meaning of sex and its function in life. Sex can be seen simply as a means of fulfilling an intimate physical need, or as the physical manifestation of the spiritual culmination in the emotional relationship between two people. During the 1980s an American lay midwife (unqualified birth attendant), Ina May Gaskin, expounded the sexual joys of childbirth and its effects on relationships. Ina May still works in a commune in Tennessee, where the birth of a baby is viewed very much as a part of the overall spiritual (and sexual) experience of individuals, couples, families and communities. The very fact that you and your partner have created this new baby, usually in a loving encounter, confirms it as a sexual experience. Your sexual organs have been changing and developing to fulfil their ultimate purpose, growing and birthing your baby and feeding and nourishing him before and afterwards. During birth, your most intimate centres will be exposed, both literally and metaphorically, and the spiritual impact which birth has on many people can have the same emotional and chemical effect as a sexual experience. Whether or not you and your partner view birth as something sexual, you will definitely be amazed by what happens to you. The sense of achievement and responsibility is awesome and you will experience the most profound feelings you may ever encounter.

Choosing who to have with you in labour

You need to give some consideration to whom you would like with you in labour – if you are in your own home, you can have as many people as you wish, but most hospitals and birth centres have a limit of two people to accompany you in the labour room, mainly for practical and logistical reasons. You should discuss with your partner, if you have one, whether he or she wishes to be with you – but try not to make him feel that he has to be there. Most men find it quite difficult to be with their partners throughout labour, mainly because it can be upsetting to see someone they love in pain, but perhaps also because they do not know what to do or how to behave and feel helpless. Some of the intimate examinations and procedures such as being stitched after the birth can also cause both partners to feel uncomfortable and embarrassed. He may want to be there emotionally but when faced with the reality of the situation he may change his mind. However, there is plenty that your partner can do to make you feel better supported and physically and emotionally comfortable during the long first stage (see Chapter 9). He may, of course, make a decision during your pregnancy not to stay for the actual birth, although very often partners find that they get caught up in the event and enjoy being present for the birth.

You may prefer to have your mother or sister or a friend with you instead. This can be comforting but do not assume that, just because your birth supporter is a woman, she will feel completely detached from the experience – if she is close enough to be with you in labour she may also experience feelings similar to those of your partner, such as anxiety, concern or embarrassment. It is as important to prepare your friend or female family member as it is to prepare your partner. It is also wise to arrange someone else as a substitute in case your first choice of companion is either unavailable or prefers not to be with you on the day – or you may change your mind when you go into labour.

Some parents decide to include their other children, the siblings of the new baby, to be present at the birth. This is very much an individual decision between you and your partner and may be dependent on your children's ages, personalities and their interest in learning about birth. A child should only be encouraged to be present if s/he wants to be there – forcing children to be in the room against their wishes may lead to a variety of psychological and relationship problems in the future. However much you feel it is what you would like, this is not about you and, for the sake of your child, do think about it very carefully. The child should be well prepared from relatively early in your pregnancy and should also be able to change his/her mind – sometimes more than once – about whether or not to be with you, and whether to remain in the room for the duration of your labour. This is not normally a problem if you are in your own home, although you should ensure that someone has been allocated to care for him/her if s/he does not want to stay there. This is particularly important in the hospital – you will probably need to request permission for your child to be with you, and will need to consider what would happen in the event of an emergency.

'Eleanor and Gary wanted to have Jessie with them during Phoebe's birth, but I wasn't very sure it would be a good thing for her. I must say they spent a lot of time talking to her beforehand and when the day came, she just ran in and out occasionally, but spent most of the day playing in the garden. Eleanor had a long labour so I suppose it was all a bit boring for Jessie. By the time Phoebe was actually born, it was nearly midnight and Jessie was asleep, so we left her until the morning to tell her the news and she was fine.'

Catherine, grandmother to Jessie, 5, and Phoebe, 7 months

In the UK and most of Europe, the majority of maternity care is provided by midwives and/or doctors. In the UK, the midwife is the 'lead professional' responsible for 70 per cent of pregnancies and births. Indeed, it is illegal for anyone other than a midwife or doctor, or one in training under supervision, to take sole responsibility for maternity care, except in an emergency. There are some male midwives too, (they are still called midwives, as the term 'mid – wife' means 'with woman' – i.e. *you*). If you prefer not to be cared for by a man, you do have the right to decline and to request a female midwife or obstetrician.

In the USA, the system differs in each state: in many states
maternity nurses work in association with medical staff but do
not have the same responsibilities as midwives in the UK and
Europe; in a few states there is a system of 'lay' midwives –
unqualified, but highly experienced women who can provide
care throughout your pregnancy and the birth. In many other
countries such as South Africa, if you are receiving private
maternity care, the doctor monitors and treats you throughout,
with midwives assisting in labour as needed, although there are
increasing numbers of private midwives who provide home birth
services.

The following table gives a summary of the roles and
responsibilities of maternity health professionals who may be
involved in caring for you during pregnancy, labour and after the
birth. It is also worth considering additional companions who are
not currently members of the conventional maternity care team.
There is a growing body of research evidence to suggest that
having a female supporter with you continuously during labour
facilitates more normal progress, helps you to work better with the
contractions and may result in a more normal birth than if you are
left alone. Instead of having a friend with you, you may choose to
hire a doula or complementary therapist to accompany you
during labour, either in addition to, or instead of your partner.

Professionals involved in maternity care

Health professional	Responsibilities
Midwife	▶ Expert in care of mothers with normal, uncomplicated pregnancies.
	▶ Delivers approximately 70 per cent of babies in UK.
	▶ Provides care for you and your baby for up to 28 days after the birth.
	▶ Works in NHS hospitals, local health centres and in your own home or may be employed by private maternity hospitals.
	▶ May be self-employed, working independently or in partnership with other midwives: you employ and pay her/him directly to provide care throughout, usually planning to have your baby at home.
Obstetrician/ gynaecologist	▶ Doctor with additional training, specializing in caring for women with complications in pregnancy or labour (hospital-based).
	▶ Usually combines maternity care with gynaecology (general women's health medicine and surgery).
	▶ Junior doctors training to become obstetricians work under the supervision of both senior obstetricians and experienced midwives.
General practitioner	▶ Works alongside midwives and obstetricians but is not qualified to provide care when complications occur except in an emergency.

(Contd)

	▶ May provide some antenatal care, monitoring your health and that of your baby during pregnancy; will usually visit you at home after the birth, but is rarely involved in the actual birth.
Paediatrician	▶ Specialist hospital doctor who cares for babies and children.
	▶ Some specialize further in neonatology, caring for sick newborn babies who are admitted to the neonatal intensive care unit.
Anaesthetist	▶ Specialist hospital doctor who is responsible for anaesthesia if you require a Caesarean or other operation.
	▶ Will insert epidural or spinal anaesthesia if you choose this.
	▶ Some specialize in pain management and may use acupuncture.
Health visitor	▶ Specially trained nurse (may also be qualified midwife), who specializes in caring for families in the local community.
	▶ Sometimes sees you during pregnancy but is mainly responsible for ensuring that you are coping with parenthood and that your baby/child is developing and growing normally.
	▶ Also provides specialist help for families with special needs, often working alongside social workers.
Maternity assistant	▶ Assists midwives and doctors with basic physical care of mothers and new babies, during pregnancy, labour and after delivery.

Health professional	Responsibilities
	▶ Works in hospital and community.
Obstetric ultrasonographer	▶ Performs ultrasound scans of your baby during pregnancy.
	▶ May also be qualified midwife able to interpret the scans and discuss with you any issues arising from them.

'I had such a long labour and so many midwives looking after me during Will's birth that I couldn't bear the thought of that again so I've booked an independent midwife for this baby. She comes to my house for all my appointments, I can phone her whenever I have a question or worry and she has really become a friend of the family now.'

Ursula, 37, now 26 weeks pregnant and planning a home birth for her second baby

DOULA

The word 'doula' comes from the Greek, meaning 'carer or female servant', but is now used to define an experienced labour companion, usually a woman who has had children of her own, who provides continuous emotional support and assistance before, during and after the birth of your baby. Their role is not to provide clinical care, such as monitoring your progress or delivering the baby, but to offer emotional and practical support, to act as your advocate and to be a source of communication between you and the professional maternity team.

If you are considering hiring a doula to accompany you in labour, you need to find one who is adequately trained to provide the range of care you need and it is important to meet with her in advance to ensure that she is someone to whom you can relate. Some doulas use a range of complementary therapies when caring for labouring mothers, but check the extent to which they have been trained to use these; you may prefer to hire someone who is a dedicated Birth Support Therapist with complementary therapy training specifically for childbirth (see Taking it further). When selecting a doula, ask how long she has been working in this role and how many families she has attended – reading references or testimonials from previous clients can be helpful. Obviously the doula needs also to be available for about three weeks either side of your due date, to ensure that she can be with you, although bear in mind that she could be attending another mother if you go into labour especially early or very much after your date; check whether she has someone who can replace her if she is busy elsewhere.

Insight

It has become popular in the USA and UK for some mothers to choose to give birth without professional help – 'free birthing' or 'unassisted birthing'. While this is not illegal (so long as no one assists) it is unwise because problems can occur very quickly if not recognized in the early stages. You are advised not to appoint a doula as your sole semi-professional assistant for your baby's birth.

There is a huge contemporary increase in the popularity of doulas in the USA, and more recently in the UK, where financial and staff constraints have adversely affected the numbers of available midwives. It is vital, however, to determine whether the doula has professional indemnity insurance cover as it is not currently a legal requirement for doulas or therapists to have insurance and there is no national mandatory registration system to check qualifications and experience (although this is in the process of changing). It would be wise also to ask for a written contract which details what the doula does and does not offer and what happens in the event of her not being able to be with you. Also ask what would happen if you change your mind and decide not to have a doula with you in labour – to what extent are you committed to paying for her services?

COMPLEMENTARY THERAPIST

You may already have used complementary therapies before becoming pregnant, or you may wish to use them to help you relax and provide alternative ways of coping with pregnancy discomforts. If you have not previously received treatment from a therapist but would like one to be with you in labour, it is important to find a well qualified, insured practitioner who is experienced in caring for pregnant and/or labouring mothers. Don't rely on the Yellow Pages to find someone – 'word of mouth' is always a good recommendation or you could ask your midwife or doctor if they can suggest someone locally. You should inform your midwife early in your pregnancy if you intend to have someone with you in labour as most maternity services will require the therapist to confirm that they have professional indemnity insurance cover; she may also be asked to sign a disclaimer form acknowledging that the midwife and/or doctor retains overall responsibility for your care. Some maternity units now offer therapies such as reflexology, aromatherapy, acupuncture or massage, although this is by no means universal and you may prefer to arrange for your own therapist to accompany you.

You should ensure that your birth companion is aware of your wishes for labour and is prepared to act as your advocate in the event that you are less able to make objective decisions than anticipated. It is also useful to have discussed what s/he should do in the event that you change your mind about your birth plan. It is not helpful, for example, if your partner/birth supporter insists that you refuse an epidural, because that was your original wish, when you have reached a stage where you are unable to cope with the contractions without it. If you are to have your mother or sister with you, try to talk through with them beforehand the reasons for your birth plan decisions – occasionally mothers/mothers-in-law can use your labour as an opportunity to reflect on their own birthing experiences and while it can sometimes be helpful to share these during pregnancy, it may be inappropriate when your labour is in full progress. Be clear about what exactly you would like your birth supporter to do – and anything you prefer them not to do. You do not want to be worrying about their behaviour/reactions on the day. See also Chapter 8 on how your birth companion can help you during labour.

10 THINGS TO REMEMBER

1 *This is your labour – so choose who you want with you.*

2 *If your partner truly does not wish to be in the labour room with you, do not force him – he may spontaneously change his mind later.*

3 *Whoever you choose to be with you, have another family member or friend 'on standby' in case the first person is unavailable.*

4 *If you wish your other children to be with you, think about how you can prepare them beforehand; if you are having your baby in hospital you will need to ask permission for them to attend.*

5 *The midwife is the lead professional who will care for you during labour, unless you have any medical or pregnancy-related conditions which require the doctor's input.*

6 *It is illegal for anyone other than a midwife or doctor to deliver your baby except in an emergency, so think very carefully if you are considering staying at home without professional help.*

7 *If you are considering having a doula to accompany you, check her training and insurance cover and obtain permission from the midwife, preferably in advance of your labour.*

8 *If you are planning to have a complementary therapist, or a doula who uses complementary therapies, with you during labour, check that they have appropriate training to use the therapies in labour (not just pregnancy) and that they understand their role and the need for your midwife to take responsibility for your care.*

9   *If professionals, other than the midwife or doctor, are
    involved in your care, ask for an explanation of their role.*

10 *Always ask questions so that you fully understand what
    is happening to you and your baby during labour and
    the birth.*

8

....

Work, rest and play

In this chapter you will learn:
- *about paternity leave for labour and new fatherhood*
- *how your birth partner can help you during labour.*

We know that having a baby is extremely hard work so it is important for both you and your partner to prepare physically and emotionally for the transition from pregnancy to parenthood. Aim to get as much rest as possible prior to labour, so do not arrange any events that are not essential in the last three to four weeks of your pregnancy. During labour, try to rest between contractions so that you do not become over-tired. Eating lightly and keeping hydrated with plenty of fluids will maintain your energy for the work your body needs to do, and preparing well in advance to help you cope with contractions will reduce stress, which can also be tiring (see also Chapter 9 on coping with contractions).

Your partner will probably need to make arrangements to take time off work for the birth and perhaps for a few days afterwards. Most employers are reasonably sympathetic to requests for time off, although the unpredictability of the birth can cause logistical difficulties in some jobs, especially for those who work away from home. In the UK, two weeks' paid paternity leave is now a statutory right, subject to regulations about length of time in employment and the amount of National Insurance contributions paid. However, your partner should be sure to inform his employer that he intends to take leave, by the twenty-fifth week of your pregnancy. Most other European countries offer paid paternity leave at least as favourable as that in the UK, if not better; in the USA fathers can take unpaid leave from companies with at least 50 employees, but must have worked a specified number of hours within the last year (see Chapter 4 on maternity benefits in the UK).

Insight

Your partner should, ideally, consult the human resources department at work early in your pregnancy, if there is one, or seek advice about paternity leave from the various government websites or telephone helplines. Early planning is vital to ensure that you receive all the benefits to which you are both entitled.

'It was quite unnerving towards the end – every time the phone rang at work in those last few weeks, my heart started thumping in case it was Sally going into labour. I had to plan my work so that I wouldn't have too many important meetings, because I knew I'd have to leave in a rush.'

Paul, 34, an insurance broker, married to Sally, 33, who has just had their first baby

In some cases, your partner may choose to add some of his annual leave allowance to his paternity leave entitlement – but he should recognize that this may be anything but a holiday. Being with you in labour can be as physically and emotionally draining for him as it is for you, albeit in different ways. It is just as important that he attends to his own needs while you are in labour, for example, adequate rest and sleep, food, drinks to prevent him from becoming dehydrated, especially if you are in a hospital labour ward which can be very warm, and some time in the fresh air. It can be just as gruelling an experience for your partner and he should prepare for it in the same way as he would for a day's walking or climbing.

If your partner is worried about how he will react during the labour, encourage him to become involved during the final few weeks of your pregnancy so that he also feels well prepared. While you are at home in early labour, he can join you in whatever distraction activities you choose, such as watching the television, listening to music or reading, or he may prefer to wash the car or mow the lawn until you need him. You could play board or card games together, or if you have not already done it, start writing all the envelopes for the birth notification cards. In the hospital or birthing centre let him know that it is acceptable to leave your room occasionally, such as when you are having an internal examination, even though he may only be able to wander round the car park or hospital shop or restaurant. Do not begrudge him these few moments of respite from what is, after all, an essentially female activity and try not to feel rejected or isolated. He will be much more use to you if he has been able to potter about doing what he wants and supporting you in between.

How your birth supporter can help you

Your birth supporter can help you physically by:

- *driving you to hospital/birth centre*
- *making drinks and snacks for you, and those with you, if you stay at home*
- *helping to keep you mobile and upright, walking with you or holding you during contractions*
- *massaging your back, feet, shoulders to keep you relaxed and help with pain*
- *encouraging you and physically helping you to change position*
- *assisting you in and out of the bath/shower or birthing pool; keeping water in pool topped up*
- *reminding you to breathe to avoid hyperventilating.*

They can also help by communicating information and news to yourself and to others:

- *contacting midwife/hospital/birth centre when you go into labour*
- *ensuring you have everything you need, e.g. labour bag, books, games, etc.*
- *sitting with you and providing moral support and encouragement*
- *organizing arrangements for other children*
- *listening to and interpreting what the midwives/doctors say*
- *acting as your advocate on things about which you have particular views*
- *keeping other family members informed of your progress.*

THINGS TO REMEMBER

1 *If you and your partner are well prepared for the birth you will understand more of what is happening and will feel more relaxed about the situation.*

2 *In the last weeks of pregnancy, eat well, keep well hydrated, rest and sleep properly; get some gentle exercise and take time to prepare yourself mentally for the birth and the imminent arrival of your new baby.*

3 *Make sure your partner has arranged paternity leave from work by the 25th week of your pregnancy so he can be with you and take some time off.*

4 *Ensure you know how to contact your partner or other birth companion when you go into labour.*

5 *Consider ways for your partner to prepare for labour so that he remains comfortable and at ease, e.g. drinks and snacks.*

6 *Most maternity units permit only two visitors to be with you at any time in the labour ward, so if you have more there may need to be a 'rota'.*

9

Physical well-being

In this chapter you will learn:
- *what physically happens to your body during labour and delivery*
- *self-help techniques to help you work with your contractions*
- *about conventional methods of relieving pain in labour*
- *about the power of water for labour and delivery*
- *how to cope when things are not as you expect for your labour.*

The technical term for birth is 'parturition', although we normally refer to it as 'labour' – because it is certainly hard work, possibly the hardest job you will ever have to do! Normal labour can occur any time from 37 weeks of pregnancy; before this, labour would be premature and after about 42 weeks you are considered 'overdue'. However, mothers go into labour at slightly different times, dependent on their own health and the baby's size, position and well-being.

Insight
Normal pregnancy lasts from 37 weeks to 43 weeks so do not panic if you do not give birth on your estimated due date: within these limits your baby should be fit and healthy and labour should progress normally.

So what actually causes labour – why do you not just keep on being pregnant? Towards the end of pregnancy your baby settles into a suitable position for the birth (usually head first or cephalic), which puts pressure on the cervix (neck of the uterus) to start the process of softening and opening/dilating it. Your uterus has grown from approximately the size of a pear and is now rather like an inflated balloon – once it reaches its maximum size the nerves become irritable and contractions start. If your baby is very big, or if you are expecting more than one baby, labour can start earlier than your expected date because your uterus becomes over-stretched at an earlier stage. The rise in the production of 'feel good' chemicals in your brain seems to make you more able to cope with labour: it is thought that if you are still very anxious about going into labour, your 'feel good' chemicals are not high enough and you are not yet ready. Your baby also produces chemicals in his brain and in the adrenal glands above the kidneys, which help to start labour contractions.

Powers, passages and passenger

Labour is a combination of three factors:

▶ *efficient contractions of your uterus and dilatation of your cervix – referred to as 'the powers' – these increase in length, strength and frequency as labour progresses*
▶ *the shape and size of your pelvis, which forms the bony canal through which your baby must travel – referred to as 'the passages'*
▶ *the size, position and well-being of your baby – 'the passenger' – who makes the hardest journey of his life through your pelvis.*

Insight

Uterine contractions cause the muscles to get shorter and thicker which, over a period of time, pushes down on your baby and encourages him to descend in your pelvis until he is low enough to be born.

In the last few weeks of pregnancy you will experience several changes in your body. Your baby settles into the most favourable position for birth and his movements slow down as he conserves energy. If you are having your first baby, he will normally settle into your pelvis by about 36 weeks – this reduces the upwards pressure which can cause heartburn and breathlessness, but puts pressure downwards onto your bladder and causes a return of frequency of urination. Your Braxton Hicks contractions, which have sent oxygen and food to the baby throughout pregnancy, will become stronger and can easily be mistaken for early labour. Although you will be tired and heavy, you may get a new lease of life and suddenly feel the need to start organizing things, cleaning and generally 'nesting'. Some mothers have slight diarrhoea for a few days before labour starts and occasionally the sickness you may have experienced in early pregnancy returns as the hormone levels shift.

Commonly, you may have a 'show', an increased vaginal discharge of thick, white jelly-like mucus, sometimes tinged with a pale streaking of blood – this is part of the mucus plug from the cervix and is a good sign that your body is getting ready to go into labour, although the 'show' can be repeated several times before labour actually starts. Occasionally, the bag of membranes surrounding the baby will break and clear fluid leaks out, making you wonder if you have 'wet yourself' – it is usually only a trickle and very rarely an absolute 'whoosh' of fluid. Contractions are the commonest sign that labour is starting, gradually increasing in length, strength and frequency, although sometimes it is difficult to know if you are actually in labour.

CASE STUDY

'I'd had a Caesarean last time, and with this baby I had quite uncomfortable Braxton Hicks contractions in the last few weeks of my pregnancy so when they got even worse I really thought I was in labour. The midwife came to the house to examine me but said I was not in labour, just "limbering up", and in fact I didn't go into labour for another four days.'

Anne, 31, mother of Rachel, 3 and Tim, 2 months

There are three stages of labour and the length of each stage varies according to whether it is your first baby or not. The *first* stage is from the onset of regular uterine contractions until your cervix is fully dilated and can last up to 24 hours, although it is normally completed within 12–18 hours. There is sometimes a short transition stage just before the birth, as the cervix finishes dilating, during which you may feel an increasing urge to bear down. The *second* stage – the birth – is from full cervical dilatation until your baby has been completely delivered and usually lasts between 30 minutes and two hours. The *third* stage involves delivery of the placenta and control of (maternal) bleeding and usually lasts between five and 45 minutes, depending on whether or not you have an injection to speed up the process.

The contractions of the first stage occur as a result of the muscles of the uterus shortening and thickening which helps to push downwards on the baby as he starts his journey to the outside world. They also assist in pulling up and opening out (dilating) the cervix or neck of the uterus, in much the same way as pulling the top of a sock up your calf. Initially, contractions feel rather like period pain, either in your back or across the top of your pubic bone, and gradually change to a tightening across your whole abdomen; indeed, the top of your abdomen will become very firm and hard as the contractions increase in intensity. Backache is common especially if your baby is lying with his back against yours (posterior position) but you may also feel discomfort in your thighs and down your legs, across your shoulders and between and under your shoulder blades and ribs. However, this discomfort usually subsides completely between contractions, allowing you time to draw breath and rest. Towards the end of the first stage of labour the contractions will probably be lasting about 60 seconds each and coming every two to three minutes.

Insight

There is an astounding difference between the discomfort you may feel during a contraction and the complete absence of sensation between contractions as your body rests and the muscles relax.

If all is well, you will be looked after by a midwife, who remains responsible for your care throughout the labour, even if complications arise and you require medical attention. In the UK it is illegal for anyone other than a midwife or doctor to deliver a baby unless it is an emergency situation. Obviously, if you are in the middle of the shopping centre and your waters break, you will be pleased for anyone around to help you, but it is not permitted for anyone else to *plan* to deliver your baby without the attendance of a midwife (this includes your partner). There have actually been one or two prosecutions of men who have delivered their partner's baby in cases where a couple has actively rejected professional care.

The aim of labour care is to ensure that you have as safe and satisfying an experience as possible, that your health and that of your baby are satisfactory and that labour progresses normally. The midwife will regularly assess your progress and well-being to ensure that you and your baby are coping. She may suggest periodic internal examinations to identify how far your labour has progressed and the position of your baby. The midwife (or your doula or therapist) will also help you to stay calm and to cope with the contractions and ensure that both you and your partner/birth supporter are comfortable, aware of and understand any developments and that you are happy with the care you are receiving.

Transition is the short period between the first and second stages of labour, in which the contractions usually increase in intensity, although sometimes they slow down temporarily as your body prepares for the final hurdle of the birth. You may feel desperately that you want to push (bear down) but the midwife may advise you not to do so if you can avoid it because the cervix may not yet be completely dilated. Sometimes a very small, irregular section of cervix remains – called a 'lip' of cervix – and this must finally open up before you can start the task of birthing your baby. It is a time when many mothers become distressed and irritable, blaming their partners for getting them pregnant, perhaps screaming, crying, shouting or swearing and saying that they 'have had enough'. Your breathing will also start to change and you may be grunting or panting – many midwives are able to assess that you are in this stage of labour even when they are outside the door of your room! Try not to worry about how you will behave at this time – midwives and doctors have seen every type of reaction to labour and this behaviour is considered a good sign of progress and imminent delivery.

The second stage of labour is the time when your baby is born. The contractions change to become very strong and expulsive but they may become more spaced apart. Passage through the birth canal is actually a series of passive movements by your baby, helped by your involuntary pushing, which causes downwards pressure of your diaphragm onto your baby's head and pushes him down towards your pelvic floor muscles. The hardest part of the second stage is pushing out your baby's head – this can take some time as the baby takes two steps forwards and one step back until he has descended far enough to come through your vagina and stretch the perineum. This can cause a stinging, burning and tearing feeling but is quite normal. Initially, your midwife may encourage you to push with each contraction but once your baby's head is almost out she will probably ask you to pant/breathe deeply to avoid pushing him out too quickly which can cause unnatural tearing of your perineum. There is sometimes a pause after his head is born – your partner may be able to see him turn to one side as he lines up his shoulders with your pelvic bones – then the rest of his body will follow naturally. Incredibly, the pain of labour stops immediately and, if all is well you should be able to enjoy holding your new baby in your arms, if you wish.

Insight

Do not worry if your baby looks blue or fails to cry immediately after he is born. During labour, there is naturally a slight reduction in oxygen to the baby, which increases his carbon dioxide levels: this is necessary because rising carbon dioxide will trigger his breathing mechanisms and make him attempt to draw breath as he is delivered.

'I couldn't believe how immediately the pain of the contractions went away once Joe's head was out. The midwife had asked me if I wanted to find out the baby's sex for myself and as he came out I could just see that he was a boy. I started crying tears of pure joy and felt this overwhelming need to hold him. It didn't matter that the placenta took another 25 minutes to come out.'

Lucy, 35, mother to Joe, now 6 months old

After your baby's birth, if you have decided to have a fairly quick third stage, you will be given an injection of artificial hormone (synthetic oxytocin, see below), which makes your uterus contract one last time. The effect of this contraction is to cause the placenta to separate from the lining of your uterus and to squeeze all the fibres of the uterine muscles so that they clamp down around the ends of the open blood vessels, to prevent you from bleeding excessively. If the hormone injection has been given, this stage takes only about five minutes but if you have decided to have a natural third stage it may take up to 45 minutes for your uterus to contract again spontaneously. Once the midwife is sure that the placenta has separated completely, it can then be delivered, either by you pushing it out or by the midwife pulling it out. The placenta is checked afterwards to ensure that it is complete and that no pieces have been left behind in your uterus, which could increase the risk of haemorrhage. Your body's clotting mechanism is also set in motion at this time to prevent major haemorrhage, although some bleeding, up to about 500 ml, is normal. Occasionally, more severe bleeding occurs and you would then need to be given an(other) injection of the hormone to make the uterus contract strongly enough to control the haemorrhage.

Your baby is dried and wrapped and the midwife will ensure he is breathing and immediately adapting to life in the outside world – a special scoring system, the APGAR score, is used in which the midwife assesses the baby's breathing, heart rate, colour, muscle tone and reaction to stimulation, such as being handled. The scoring system is marked out of ten, two marks for each category. The normal APGAR score is about 9/10 as most babies 'lose' one mark because their hands and feet are slightly blue until their circulation has adapted sufficiently to push oxygen round the body fully.

Your midwife will help you to change out of soiled clothing and bed sheets and make sure that you have recovered from the immediate effects of the delivery. She will then help you to fix your new baby on the breast if you are intending to breastfeed, or help you to position him for his first bottle-feed, and will bring you and your partner a wonderfully welcome and refreshing cup of tea or coffee. Unless there are any problems, you will probably be left together for a while so you can get to know your baby. A little later the midwife will return to check your blood pressure, blood loss, whether you need stitches and to help you shower or bathe, as well as examining your baby to make sure everything is normal, before either leaving you with your family if you are at home or transferring you to the post-natal ward if you are in hospital. In the UK it is a legal requirement that the midwife remains with you for at least one hour after delivery (often called the *fourth* stage of labour), although in reality it is usually much longer than this before everything has been sorted.

Working with contractions

Labour is almost always painful, due to muscle contractions in your uterus, which are the transmission of sensations along nerve pathways to your brain and the impact of various chemicals in the brain. It is *natural*, physiological pain and is not a result of disease or illness, which causes unnatural or pathological pain. Labour also allows you a period of mental adjustment as you realize that your pregnancy is almost over and that you are going to become a parent – surprisingly, those few mothers who have a pain-free labour often feel that they have missed out and that the transition from being pregnant to being a parent is too sudden. The extent to which you will feel pain during your labour is influenced by your personal perception, based on your personality and your attitude to labour and the arrival of your baby. Various factors, both positive and negative, can affect your perception of the pain, including how prepared, in control and well supported you feel, fear and anxiety about the anticipated pain, previous experiences of pain, cultural perspectives, concern about either your own or your baby's health, as well as existing illness or the development of problems during labour. You need to work with the pain rather than fight against it – think of it as a means to an end, with every contraction bringing you closer to meeting your baby.

One of the most important hormones involved in labour is oxytocin, produced from the pituitary gland in your brain, which also plays a part in sexual intercourse and in breastfeeding. During sex, oxytocin enhances ovulation (and, in men, increases sperm production) to facilitate conception, causes uterine contractions during orgasm and triggers the cervix to suck in the semen to meet the egg and, in conjunction with other hormones, makes you feel good afterwards. In pregnancy, the oxytocin enables good blood flow to the placenta and your baby through the Braxton Hicks contractions. During labour, oxytocin stimulates the onset of contractions in your uterus and, in the second stage, also facilitates relaxation of the muscles of the pelvic floor and vaginal walls to allow space for your baby to be delivered. It helps to control haemorrhage by contracting your uterus and, later, aids the return of your uterus to its non-pregnant size, shape and position. After delivery, oxytocin plays a part in lactation by contracting special cells surrounding the milk cells, thereby helping to eject milk into your baby's mouth.

Other chemicals – endorphins – also need to be released to aid labour progress. Endorphins are naturally occurring, pain-relieving chemicals and act as your body's 'feel good' factors. They appear to have a slightly amnesiac property, perhaps helping you to forget the worst of the pain in a previous labour so that you can approach a subsequent birth without that memory. However, endorphins are released in response to pain, so in order to be produced in sufficient quantities, it is necessary first to feel the pain of early labour contractions. This is why, if you have labour induced, it is inappropriate to have an epidural or spinal anaesthetic before adequate contractions are established since insufficient endorphins are produced. This could adversely affect labour progress and, later, leave you with a sense of depression and dissatisfaction, which could affect your relationship with your new baby.

Oxytocin release in labour can be affected by fear and anxiety as well as other negative emotions such as embarrassment. Unresolved psychological and emotional issues related to previous experiences, such as excessive pain or complications in your last labour, or more profound issues such as sexual abuse, can prevent adequate oxytocin release. Unfortunately, fear of anticipated pain in labour can trigger some of the endorphins to be produced prematurely in an attempt to make you feel better, but this in turn inhibits the release of oxytocin so that your contractions do not become powerful enough to trigger sufficient beneficial endorphins to subdue the pain. This sets up a negative cycle of events – see Figure 9.1.

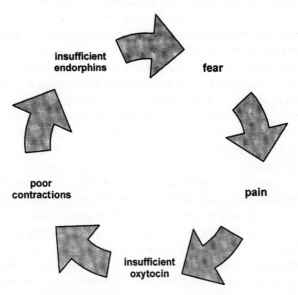

insufficient
endorphins

fear

poor
contractions

pain

insufficient
oxytocin

Figure 9.1 The fear of anticipated pain in labour.

It is therefore important to try to reduce any anxieties you have about your labour by finding out as much as you can beforehand and preparing mentally for the work to come. Oxytocin production is also affected by the use of some drugs, including anaesthetics, which interfere with oxytocin-sensitive areas in the body. Inadequate release of oxytocin leads to a more prolonged labour and may increase the chance of needing intervention to speed up your labour and of having an instrumental delivery such as a forceps or Caesarean section. It also increases the risks of excessive haemorrhage after the birth of your baby because there is inadequate uterine contraction to shut off the blood vessels. This is why it is necessary to ensure that you are as fit and healthy as possible during pregnancy to facilitate good progress in labour.

Insight

Remember that stress hormones interfere with the release of labour hormones. There is a fine balance between the two types of hormones, therefore keeping calm can contribute to a more efficient labour and better progress towards the birth.

If your labour progresses normally, it is easier to cope with the contractions than if problems develop, when you may need stronger pain relief such as an epidural. However, if this becomes necessary, stay positive and tell yourself that you have done the best you can and it is now time to ask for something more to help you. It is much better if you have help to cope with the pain so that your labour remains as near normal as possible – trying to 'soldier on' with what may seem to you to be unbearable pain can sometimes lead to other complications because it reduces both the oxytocin and the endorphins so necessary to good progress. If you are sensitive to the way your body works, stronger pain relief can accomplish the task much more quickly and efficiently.

Top tip

Deal with one contraction at a time. Labour pain is normal and quite different from the pain of disease or injury – your body is designed to cope with it and it is necessary to help you progress towards a normal labour and birth.

During pregnancy, ask your midwife or doctor to clarify anything you do not understand. If a partner or friend is going to accompany you during labour, ask him/her to be prepared to act as your advocate, taking your wishes into account, even when you are not in a fit state to be assertive yourself. If you are due to have your baby in hospital, stay at home as long as you feel reasonably comfortable – if you go into the maternity unit too early, you will have only your contractions to think about and this will make them seem more painful. Also, there is a tendency for some midwives and doctors to feel that they must 'do something' once you are in the labour ward, which may mean you are advised to have your labour speeded up sooner than might have been the case had you stayed at home.

SELF-HELP TECHNIQUES FOR WORKING WITH CONTRACTIONS

Technique	How to use
Aromatherapy	• Essential oils used in the bath or in massage can ease pain, anxiety and nausea and may aid contractions.
Bach flower remedies	• Rescue Remedy may reduce stress (four drops) – good for your partner too, especially if he panics! • Try olive for tiredness and mimulus for fear – two drops of each, neat on your tongue or in water.
Birthing ball	• Use a birthing ball on which you can sit astride – this helps you get into a comfortable position and is more favourable to the progress of labour.
Breathing	• Try to avoid breathing too heavily during contractions as this can make you feel dizzy and light-headed. • Sigh Out Slowly (SOS) – focus on breathing out by exhaling with a big 'sigh of relief', letting breathing in take care of itself – you will not forget to breathe in, just try not to concentrate on it.
Comfort	• Stay cool – wear an old T-shirt and tracksuit bottoms. • Keep paper knickers ready for when your bag of waters has broken. • Use a fan and a facial spray to keep you cool and refreshed.

(Contd)

- A hot water bottle (covered) or a gel pad heated in the microwave can be good to press against painful areas, e.g. lower back (take care not to burn your skin).
- Warm socks will prevent your feet from getting cold (common).

Homeopathic remedies Use 30C strength – one tablet every 15 minutes as appropriate. Inform your midwife you are taking remedies.

- *Aconite*: if your contractions are rapid; you have backache, headache, feel faint, cannot stand noise or fear your baby may die.
- *Caulophyllum*: if you have short, irregular, distressing contractions; pain down legs and groin; flying in all directions; feel exhausted, nauseous; worse when cold.
- *Chamomilla*: if you have unbearable, spasmodic contractions; back pain; sweating; thirst; are rude; nervous; exhausted; 'can't bear it any more'.
- *Cimicifuga*: if you have strong contractions which slow down when you are hot; you are hysterical; talk constantly; cannot stand noise; have a fear of the actual delivery and of dying.
- *Lycopodium*: if you have spasmodic upwards contractions; are anxious; crying; restless; press your feet against bed; feel better if you move around.
- *Gelsemium*: if you have contractions which radiate to your thighs, back and hips; have a headache; look dark and flushed; feel exhausted; sick; feel better if you bend forwards.

- *Pulsatilla*: if you have distressing, changeable ineffective contractions moving left to right and back; are apologetic; need sympathy; look pale; feel nauseous; have a dry mouth.
- *Sepia*: if you have contractions which shoot upwards into your back; feel as if there is a ball in your rectum; feel better if you cross your legs; are irritable, indifferent and resentful; have cold extremities.

Hypnotherapy

- Learn self-hypnosis during pregnancy to relax you and to block out specific fears or anxieties about labour and birth.
- Consult a hypnotherapist or buy CDs (see Taking it further).
- You will usually be taught trigger words for self-hypnosis in labour.

Massage

- Ask your companion to massage your feet, shoulders and 'bump'.
- Massage in the small of your back. Using a firm touch with the heel of the hand is best and applies most pressure.
- A very light clockwise abdominal massage during contractions may relieve pain.
- Shoulder massage eases stiffness.
- Foot massage warms your feet and aids circulation.

Mobility

- Keep upright and mobile.
- Try standing, sitting, leaning against a wall, over a chair, on all fours.

(Contd)

Technique	How to use
	• Avoid lying down for as long as possible – this may slow down labour and makes you feel much more like an 'ill patient'.
Shiatsu	• Pressure applied intermittently to acupuncture points can be pain-relieving – your partner can do this for you during each contraction. • These points are in the 'dimples' about 1–2 cm either side of your spine in the small of your back (see Figure 9.2).
Other therapies	• It may be possible to have a private therapist with you in labour for acupuncture or reflexology. • Check with your midwife antenatally – do not leave it till the last minute.
Water	• A warm bath is relaxing, eases pain and discomfort, especially if the water is deep enough to cover your 'bump'. • Make sure you are not alone in the house and that you can get out of the bath easily when you need to.

Conventional methods of relieving labour pain

For many women using some of the self-help suggestions above may be sufficient to help them through the first stage of labour, but others sometimes need stronger pain relief to help them to cope. Remember – this is *your* experience, nobody else's – and only you can say how you feel at the time. If you get to the stage in your labour where self-help suggestions are not enough for you, or if your labour is prolonged or complicated, you may need

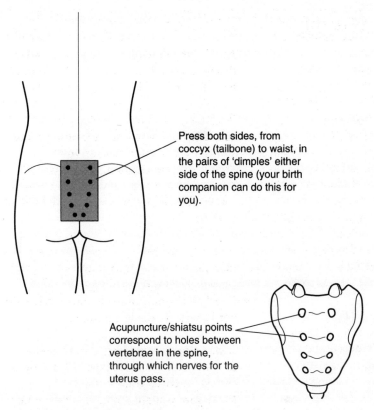

Press both sides, from coccyx (tailbone) to waist, in the pairs of 'dimples' either side of the spine (your birth companion can do this for you).

Acupuncture/shiatsu points correspond to holes between vertebrae in the spine, through which nerves for the uterus pass.

Figure 9.2 Shiatsu points to relieve pain in labour.

something else to help you cope. Do not feel let down or guilty about this – it is important that you make this decision for yourself in order to stay in control of what is happening. In no way does it mean that you have somehow 'failed' if you use drugs or have an epidural to help you – regard this as a positive move for your baby. If you reject additional pain relief when you need it, you will become tired and distressed, labour will become prolonged because the oxytocin and endorphin levels will be affected and you will feel less able to enjoy welcoming your baby when he is born.

There are several options that may be offered to you, although it may depend on where you choose to have your baby as to whether all forms of pain relief are available. For example, it is not possible to have an epidural if you are at home and this will need to be taken into account when deciding on your preferred place of birth.

ENTONOX™

Entonox™ – 50 per cent nitrous oxide (laughing gas) and 50 per cent oxygen – can be given either via a mask over your mouth and nose or, more commonly, via a mouthpiece. Entonox™ is available in maternity units and birth centres and a small portable cylinder can be used if you have your baby at home. It is helpful for just 'taking the edge off' the pain but is unlikely to relieve it completely; therefore, if you start using this in early labour, you may need stronger pain relief as labour progresses. It can also make you feel slightly disorientated and nauseous and make your mouth dry, while the nitrous oxide can make you giggle if you use it for a long time.

TENS

Transcutaneous electrical nerve stimulation (TENS) is available in many maternity units; you can also hire the equipment privately (see Taking it further). TENS is the use of pulsed electrical stimulation via small rubber pads placed on your back over areas where the nerves to your uterus pass, about an inch either side of your spine, at the level of your waist (see Figure 9.3). The pads are attached to wires connected to a small box, which enables you to adjust the amount of pulsation you require to relieve pain. TENS works on a principle similar to acupuncture, in which touch impulses reach the brain quicker than pain impulses; it also triggers the release from your brain of pain relieving and 'feel good' chemicals. It is best to start using TENS early in your labour as it can take some time to build up and become effective. The big advantage of TENS is that it appears to have no adverse effects on your labour or your baby and enables you to remain in control, although conversely, it does not always provide sufficient pain relief.

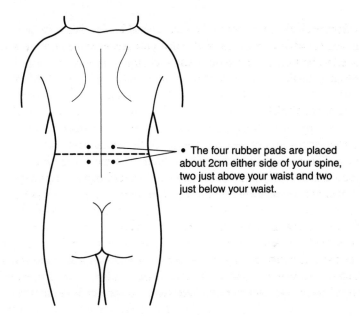

The four rubber pads are placed about 2cm either side of your spine, two just above your waist and two just below your waist.

Figure 9.3 Location of rubber pads for TENS maching in labour.

Caution: if you obtain access to a TENS machine before about 37 weeks of pregnancy, you should not use it until you are actually in labour as some research has suggested that it can trigger premature labour, leading to possible complications. Also, if you are considering a water birth, you will not be able to use TENS once you are immersed in the birthing pool.

Injections of pain relieving drugs, such as pethidine, a morphine-like drug, or meptazinol, can help to make you feel more comfortable, especially if all you need is a boost towards the end of the first stage of labour until it is time for you to push your baby out. These are quite effective painkillers, with the newer meptazinol (Meptid™) considered to be more effective than pethidine, although it is not available in all maternity units. However, either of these drugs can make you feel sick (meptazinol is possibly worse) so they are usually given with another drug to combat this. The drug may also make you feel light-headed and out of control, although this tends to happen only when you have had several doses. One of the main disadvantages of pethidine is that it can cause your baby to be slow to breathe if it is given too close to the time of the actual birth, because it passes through the placenta to your baby. The midwife will need to assess the progress of your labour, probably by internal examination, before giving you the injection. In the event of rapid progress to the delivery, your baby can be given a small injection to reverse the effects, but he may continue to be sleepy for a few days. The effects of meptazinol on the baby appear to be less problematic, with his APGAR score at birth generally being higher than those whose mothers received pethidine in labour.

EPIDURAL

Epidural or spinal anaesthetic is a local anaesthetic injection given into your lower back by the doctor (anaesthetist). After giving you a small injection to numb the area, a large needle is inserted through the skin of your back into the space between two of your spinal bones until it reaches the part of your spinal canal where the nerve endings for the uterus are situated (see Figure 9.4). A fine tube is passed down the needle and left in your back and the needle is removed. The specific painkilling drug is injected to work directly on the nerves to reduce pain. This is 'topped up' by your midwife as you need it or may be given through a continuous pump. Epidurals are especially good if you have a long, tiring labour – being pain-free allows you to sleep – or if you need a Caesarean section. You may also be advised to consider an epidural if you are in premature labour or if there are other complications, as complete pain relief can enable your body to do its work without the stress of progressive discomfort. You would, however, be advised against having an epidural if you have any blood clotting disorders, an infection such as severe genital herpes, very low blood pressure or, occasionally, major back problems. The epidural drug can cause a drop in blood pressure so you will automatically be given an intravenous drip to replace fluid if necessary, and your contractions and your baby's heartbeat will be monitored with a cardiotocograph machine. Some units offer 'mobile epidurals' so that you can be up and about in labour, although the dose of the drug used tends to be smaller so it may not be quite as effective as the normal type.

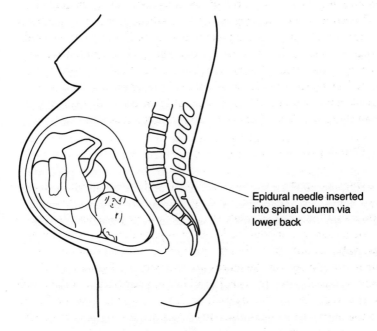

Figure 9.4 Location of epidural anaesthetic for pain relief in labour.

Epidurals can sometimes cause difficulties with passing urine so you may require a catheter to be inserted, with an increased risk of urinary infection. There is a slightly higher risk of forceps delivery as the loss of sensation caused by the epidural can mean that you are unable to feel where to push your baby out for the birth. A few mothers suffer headaches, neck or backache in the first few days after delivery but this usually passes off fairly quickly. Very occasionally, the procedure of inserting the needle into your back can cause it to move too far inwards, causing what is called a 'dural tap', leading to severe headaches and requiring you to lie flat for 24 hours to recover. More severe complications are, fortunately, very rare.

The power of water

Water can offer a very pleasant and effective medium to ease discomfort in labour and some mothers choose to stay in the water until after the birth of their baby, although you would normally be advised to get out of the pool for the delivery of the placenta, as it is necessary for the midwife to be able to estimate how much blood you have lost. Some maternity units and most birth centres provide water birth facilities, although their availability on the day you are in labour depends on whether any other mother is using them. It is also possible to hire a portable pool for use in the home – you may even be able to take this with you into the hospital or birth centre, but check with the staff first. If you decide to hire your own pool you need to be sure that the floor can withstand the weight of the water – if you live in a flat/apartment the floor may not be strong enough and it would therefore not be possible to have a water birth at home.

Insight

If the idea of a water birth appeals to you and your partner you may be able to attend water birth preparation classes; however, do not be disappointed if you change your mind about using the birthing pool once you are in labour.
Do not feel committed to using it just because you have planned/paid for it.

LABOUR AND BIRTH IN WATER

Advantages
- *It aids relaxation and comfort.*
- *You can move about easily.*
- *You feel more in control.*
- *Pain is reduced and fewer pain relieving drugs may be needed.*
- *The length of labour may be less.*
- *Your blood pressure is reduced.*
- *There is less chance of forceps/Caesarean.*
- *There is less chance of stitches after birth.*

Disadvantages
- *Water may slow down contractions.*
- *Water may increase your temperature and reduce the oxygen supply to the baby.*
- *Baby may inhale water (rare).*
- *Baby may become cold quickly.*
- *There is an increased risk of jaundice in baby.*
- *It is difficult to assess your blood loss.*

Suitability for a water birth
- *You should be 37+ weeks pregnant.*
- *You need to be expecting only one baby.*
- *You should have no medical or pregnancy complications.*
- *Your labour must progress normally.*

Reasons why you may not be able/wish to have a water birth
- *If you are in premature labour before 37 weeks.*
- *If you are suffering from an infection, e.g. hepatitis B, C or HIV.*
- *If you require epidural pain relief.*
- *If complications arise during labour.*
- *You may not feel comfortable in water.*

'My friend had her baby in water and I thought that sounded quite nice. I talked to the midwife at the hospital and she said they didn't have a special birthing pool but I could hire one and take it in with me. It was really lovely to be in the water during the first stage but I wanted to get out when Oliver was about to be born and I was on all fours by the side of the pool for his actual birth.'

Pat, 36, mother to Oliver, three weeks old

CASE STUDY

How to cope when things are not as you expect

Occasionally, despite every effort to ensure that you are in good health for your baby's birth, complications arise, either in pregnancy or during labour, which require medical attention to ensure that you and your baby remain safe and well. If you already have a medical condition that may affect your pregnancy or labour, you will be advised to have a variety of tests, investigations and treatment which aim to minimize the complications and effects on you and your baby. If problems develop during pregnancy, you can still prepare for your baby's birth, despite perhaps having to change your initial plans for labour. Complications that occur during labour can be the most disappointing, as they may mean that you cannot achieve the birth you had wished for, but try to remain positive by appreciating that the problems have been recognized and steps have been taken to solve them. Whatever your wishes for your labour, you will want your baby to be as fit and healthy as possible and in the event of unforeseen circumstances, you will want all the professional help that is available.

Try not to worry as most problems can be recognized during pregnancy or as they are beginning to develop in labour, before they become too serious. The purpose of having the midwife and/or doctor with you is so that they can monitor your progress in labour and try to prevent serious complications, and if treatment is necessary it can be started promptly.

Induction of labour

As we discussed earlier, it can be rather confusing when it comes to estimating your baby's due date as doctors and midwives calculate this date from the first day of your last normal menstrual period. This is because, since it is impossible for professionals to know exactly when you conceived (even if *you* do!), the only true point of reference is the first day of menstrual bleeding. However, the variable length of your cycle is not always taken into account when it comes to working out whether or not labour is overdue. Ultrasound scans are much more accurate these days but it is still not possible to be absolutely definite about the expected date of your baby's birth.

Do not rely on your due date too much but be prepared to go into labour any time between 37 and 43 weeks of pregnancy. Although it can be very frustrating to go overdue, do not rush to upset what is, after all, a natural process. On the other hand, try not to feel pressurized to have an induction of labour – many obstetricians will advise induction when you are about 10–14 days past your due date, as it is thought that the placenta (afterbirth) begins to deteriorate after this, and although your baby's growth slows down towards the end of pregnancy, continued weight gain can mean your baby is rather larger than anticipated to fit through your birth canal. Additionally, your baby's skull starts to harden up after the due date so his head may be less able to adapt to your bony pelvis. You, too, are likely to be very tired by this time and your blood pressure may increase, which is another reason for induction of labour. However, you *do* have the right to refuse induction, but try to find out as much as possible about your particular situation and ask for answers to your questions so that you can make an informed decision about whether or not to go ahead.

Sometimes the bag of waters surrounding your baby ruptures earlier than expected but contractions do not start naturally, so artificial hormones to stimulate uterine contractions and to speed up the birth are advised, as there is now an increased risk of infection reaching your baby via your vagina. If your baby's position has been very changeable, your obstetrician may advise induction at a time when your baby is in a favourable position for delivery, i.e. head first or breech, rather than lying across your uterus. If you have a medical condition, such as diabetes, heart or kidney disease, planning to deliver your baby early by inducing labour facilitates monitoring your condition to prevent complications. However, if your condition and that of your baby remain satisfactory, there is no medical reason to have labour started artificially. Blood tests, ultrasound scans and cardiotocograph (CTG) monitoring tests can be performed to check that everything is normal.

There are several methods of induction, including a membrane 'sweep' or breaking the bag of waters surrounding your baby during an internal examination by the midwife. Artificial hormones can be given vaginally in a pessary or intravenously via a drip, but the table below gives some suggestions for self-help techniques to encourage labour to start if it is appropriate to do so. Please note that many of these *should not* be started before you are at least 37 weeks pregnant and only if you have been advised to have labour induced in hospital. Do *not* try any of the suggestions if you have medical or pregnancy-related problems without first seeking advice from your midwife or doctor.

Insight

It cannot be stressed too strongly that labour and birth are natural processes which occur when you and your baby are ready. Many women read about natural methods of starting labour and just want to get everything over and done with. However, please seek advice from your midwife about any self-help methods you may wish to try. It is not appropriate to try all the self-help methods together.

SELF-HELP TECHNIQUES TO ENCOURAGE LABOUR TO START

Technique	How to use
Nipple massage	• This stimulates the oxytocin hormone to start contractions. • Massage each nipple between the forefinger and thumb – five minutes daily after 37 weeks of pregnancy. • Massage one nipple at a time to avoid excessively strong contractions.
Sex	• Stimulation of your cervix by your partner's penis causes local release of prostaglandin hormone inside your cervix. • Semen also contains prostaglandins to help trigger contractions. • Orgasm also causes uterine contractions.

Technique	How to use
	• Masturbation may have the same effect (and this can obviously be enjoyed at any time!).
Raspberry leaf tea *It is not necessary to take raspberry leaf routinely, especially if you have previously had a normal labour.*	• This tones uterine muscles, facilitating better contractions in labour. • It is usually recommended to start drinking raspberry leaf tea around 30 weeks; you could try it just before labour but it may not be successful in triggering contractions • Sip 2–3 cups of the tea daily. • Avoid raspberry leaf if you have had a previous Caesarean, need a planned Caesarean and birth this time, if you have previously had a very rapid labour, or if you or your baby have any medical problems.
Aromatherapy	• Add 4–6 drops of lavender and clary sage oil, diluted in a teaspoonful of grapeseed oil to your bath to relax you and encourage contractions. • Do not use oils if your waters have broken as they may affect your baby's eyes.
Acupressure	• There are several acupuncture points which can stimulate contractions (avoid until late pregnancy) – press each point 20–30 times intermittently. • Try Large Intestine 4, deep in the webbing between your thumb and first finger.

(Contd)

- Also try Spleen 6, a tender point three fingers up from the top of your inside ankle bone (see Figure 9.5).

Relaxing therapies

- Massage and reflexology can be very relaxing and encourage your body to go into labour naturally.
- These therapies should preferably be performed by a therapist who is also a midwife/nurse who can assess whether it is safe to treat you.

Homeopathic remedies
These need to be chosen according to your precise situation.

- *Caulophyllum*: if you are overdue; irritable; apprehensive; tired but cannot sleep; are sensitive to cold; thirsty.
- *Chamomilla*: if you cannot bear it; are difficult to please; restless; frequently passing pale urine; sensitive to noise and pain; feel faint; nauseous and have headaches and wind.
- *Cimicifuga*: if you have left-sided rheumatic type pain; talk incessantly; are frightened of labour and birth, and of going insane and of death; have cervix pain during internal examinations.
- *Pulsatilla*: if you keep crying; are apologetic; changeable and helpless; need lots of reassurance; have a dry mouth; feel nauseous; feel faint and sleepy but feel better in fresh air and when slowly moving about.

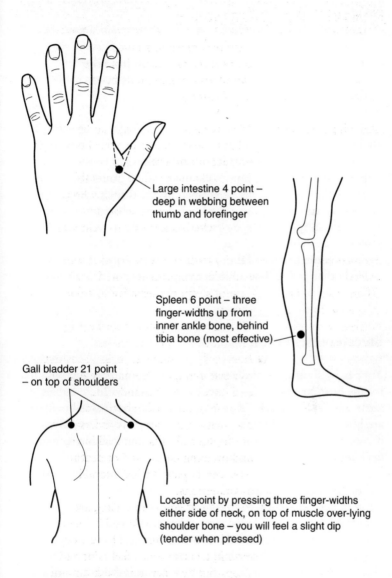

Large intestine 4 point –
deep in webbing between
thumb and forefinger

Spleen 6 point – three
finger-widths up from
inner ankle bone, behind
tibia bone (most effective)

Gall bladder 21 point
– on top of shoulders

Locate point by pressing three finger-widths
either side of neck, on top of muscle over-lying
shoulder bone – you will feel a slight dip
(tender when pressed)

All points on both sides of body – stimulate each point intermittently

Figure 9.5 Shiatsu points to stimulate contractions.

Breech presentation

Your baby should normally settle into a position that is favourable for the birth by about 34–35 weeks of pregnancy. Most babies settle into a cephalic (head-first) presentation, but occasionally they are bottom-first, or breech. This can happen if your baby is big, if your pelvis is small or a slightly different shape from normal, or if your placenta is lying low in the uterus (placenta praevia, which fills up the space where your baby's head would normally settle). Excessive fluid around your baby may mean he is more likely to keep changing position and so he could be breech when you start labour, or if there is not enough fluid he is less able to move and may get stuck in the breech position. If you have had several babies, your abdominal muscles may not be strong enough to support your baby in a position which is suitable for a normal birth, and if you are expecting twins or triplets, it is more likely that one will be breech, even if the other is head-first. A scan in late pregnancy will usually show if your baby is breech, or the midwife may feel it when she examines you at your antenatal appointment. Your baby's kicking may be lower down than expected, or you may become breathless and suffer heartburn towards the end of pregnancy, as his head pushes up under your diaphragm and compresses the base of your lungs. If you have had a breech baby before, there is an increased chance that this baby will be breech too. Very occasionally, the midwife will realize your baby is breech when she examines you internally in labour, although this is rare nowadays because scans usually detect it earlier.

Breech babies sometimes have difficulty during labour and can become distressed, so most doctors advise a Caesarean to ensure your baby is born safely, although recent research from Canada and Egypt suggests that a Caesarean for breech is only necessary when there are other medical indications. However, if your baby is discovered to be breech before you go into labour, you do have the right to try for a normal labour so that your baby can be born vaginally, although the doctor may actively attempt to discourage you. If you insist, you will normally be advised to compromise by having your baby in hospital, although the choice of place of birth remains yours. In the UK, an independent midwife will usually agree to care for you at home if you choose to pay for this service, or if you prefer NHS care and wish to stay at home, a midwife is legally required to attend you (interestingly, doctors have the right to refuse!).

A commonly offered medical treatment to try to turn the baby is external cephalic version (ECV), an abdominal procedure performed by the doctor at around 35–37 weeks of pregnancy. You are usually given an intravenous injection to relax you and the baby will be scanned to ensure he is still breech; this will also confirm the position of your placenta to ensure that it is safe to try to turn your baby. The obstetrician will then carry out an abdominal 'massage', which takes about ten minutes and should not be painful, although it can be uncomfortable. Afterwards, you and your baby will be monitored for a few hours to make sure that you are both in a satisfactory condition to go home. However, the success rate of turning babies to head-first is only about

50 per cent and complications such as fetal distress, because the baby becomes entangled in his cord, or premature labour due to stress on your uterus, can occur. Complications developing at the time of the procedure would require you to have an immediate Caesarean, so ECV is always performed in hospital. ECV is not offered if you have high blood pressure, diabetes or if you have had any bleeding in later pregnancy.

The only other medical option for breech babies is a Caesarean section (see p. 165). If you are expecting twins, and one is breech, attempts to turn him are not possible as the two babies may get tangled up together. If you have already had a baby, it will depend what the previous birth was like since some complications, such as your pelvis being too small to allow the baby through, can occur in a subsequent labour. If your placenta is lying low in the uterus, it is impossible for your baby to be born vaginally, as there is a risk that you may haemorrhage uncontrollably. If you have had assisted conception (IVF), you may not wish to risk a vaginal birth, although this may be very disappointing for you.

Moxibustion, a traditional Chinese technique to turn a breech baby to head-first, has become increasingly popular and some midwives now offer this as an alternative to ECV. It is also performed by acupuncturists, although you should try to find one who has specific experience of obstetrics. Chinese medicine is based on energy lines, called meridians, which flow around the body linking one part to another. There are numerous focus points along these meridians and one point in particular, the Bladder 67 point, on the outer edges of the little toes, is thought to link with the uterus (see Figure 9.6). Moxa sticks of dried mugwort, a herb, are used as a heat source to stimulate this point, triggering changes in the hormone levels and slightly relaxing the uterus. The baby's heart rate also increases and this, together with the extra 'give' in the uterus, helps the baby to turn to head-first. Some therapists perform the procedure for you, while others will show you what to do and send you home to do this for yourself. The treatment needs to be done for 15 minutes, twice a day, for up to ten treatments (five days), although if you think the baby has turned you should stop until you have had his position checked.

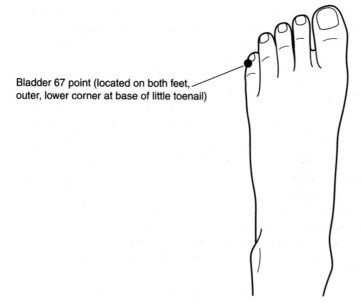

Bladder 67 point (located on both feet, outer, lower corner at base of little toenail)

Figure 9.6 Bladder 67 acupuncture point for moxibustion to turn breech baby.

'When I found out my baby was breech at 34 weeks, I panicked. I'd read about the possible risks of trying to turn the baby and I didn't want the doctor to do that. My midwife advised me to try different positions to help the baby turn, but that didn't work, so I asked her about trying moxibustion. She didn't do it herself but I was lucky to find an independent midwife locally who did offer the service so I saw her. Whatever she did, it worked and I am now hoping to have a nice normal head-first birth.'

Charlotte, 39, 38 weeks pregnant

Various research studies have shown moxibustion to be, on average, about 66 per cent successful if performed towards the end of pregnancy. One study found an extremely high success rate of 92 per cent, but as many of the mothers in this trial were only 29 or 30 weeks pregnant, it is probable that some of the babies turned back to breech – this is one of the reasons why the procedure is usually left until 34 or 35 weeks of pregnancy. There are a few reasons why moxibustion would not be appropriate or safe, similar to the reasons for not performing an ECV, so it is best to check with your midwife before consulting a practitioner who offers this service.

Top tip

Please *do not* attempt moxibustion without informing your midwife or doctor. *It is essential* to ensure that your baby is still breech before you start the procedure and, if at any time, you think he has turned, stop the moxibustion until you have had your baby's position confirmed.

Insight

You should not consider moxibustion if you have any medical or pregnancy problems or if you are due to have a planned Caesarean for a specific reason. Moxibustion is contraindicated if you have had a previous Caesarean, if you have twins, high blood pressure, a low-lying placenta (placenta praevia) or if there is excessive or insufficient fluid around the baby. If in doubt, check with your midwife.

Two homeopathic remedies which are also thought to help a breech baby to turn to head-first are pulsatilla and nux vomica (see also Part four). Pulsatilla is suitable if you keep changing your mind about what you want and it has been suggested by one American homeopathic doctor that it may be effective in turning 50 per cent of breech babies, although there is very little research on it. Natrum muriaticum is thought to regulate fluid balance and is useful if you have dry skin and lips, sluggish bowels resulting in constipation and only a small amount of fluid around your baby. Alternatively, it may also be used if you have a lot of fluid, for example oedema (swelling) in your legs, together with watery eyes, a head cold and a lot of fluid around your baby. It is best, however, to consult a homeopath before taking these remedies. Homeopathic attempts to turn your baby to head-first should not be used at the same time as any of the other methods, including moxibustion.

Chiropractic can be effective in turning a breech baby if you have lower back problems or previous injury or surgery, as this may affect the size, shape and angle of your pelvis, causing your baby to settle into an unobstructed and more comfortable position than head-first. The chiropractor uses the 'Webster technique' to manipulate your spine and related muscles to free up some space for your baby's head and allow him to turn.

Hypnotherapy has also been shown in research studies to be effective, especially if you are stressed and anxious about your baby being breech. This is because stress hormones such as adrenaline and noradrenaline reduce muscle tone, both in your uterus and in your baby, meaning that he becomes 'floppy' and is unable to hold himself in a position which is favourable for a normal birth. One research study achieved a success rate of 81 per cent using hypnosis to turn breech babies, compared to 48 per cent in a group of mothers with breech babies who had no hypnosis. Even if your baby fails to turn, hypnosis can prepare you mentally and physically for the labour by relaxing you and helping you to remain in control.

Caesarean section

The majority of mothers – about 70 per cent – have normal vaginal deliveries but occasionally assistance may be needed, such as an episiotomy, a forceps or ventouse (vacuum) delivery or a Caesarean section. An episiotomy is a cut in the perineum to enlarge the birth opening; a forceps delivery involves placing metal 'hands' around the baby's head to pull him out and a ventouse extraction is a method of instrumental delivery in which a vacuum cup is applied to the baby's skull to suck him out. A Caesarean is a major abdominal operation, which is performed when vaginal delivery is not possible, and may be elective (planned) or an emergency situation. It can be done before labour starts or at any time during the first or second stage of labour in the event of unforeseen complications. Sometimes, problems arise in late pregnancy or when you are in labour which mean that the baby has to be delivered quickly, either because he is in distress or has difficulty negotiating the birth canal, or because you become unwell before or during labour. However, if a Caesarean becomes inevitable, look on it as a positive way for your baby to be born safe and well.

There are several reasons why you may need a Caesarean section, including medical conditions such as high blood pressure, diabetes, epilepsy or heart disease, pregnancy complications, especially bleeding and vaginal infections such as herpes, if your baby is very ill, premature, too large to fit through your pelvis or not in a normal head-first position, i.e. breech or transverse, or because of labour problems, e.g. fetal distress or an excessively long labour. You will need to give consent for the operation and an anaesthetist will ensure you are fit for an anaesthetic. Your blood will be checked to make sure you are not anaemic and to reconfirm your blood group in case you need a blood transfusion. You will not be allowed to have anything to eat or drink on the day and may be given antacid medicine to stop you regurgitating acid contents from your stomach during the operation. Your abdominal and pubic hair may be shaved for hygiene purposes, although research suggests that it is not essential and not all maternity units insist on this. Your make-up, jewellery, watch and contact lenses will need to be removed beforehand (give them to someone to look after) and you may be asked to wear special thick stockings designed to prevent thrombosis (blood clots). Immediately before the anaesthetic, you will be asked to empty your bladder and you may have a catheter inserted to remove any urine during the operation.

A spinal anaesthetic or epidural inserted into your back is the most common and safest anaesthetic, with recovery being quicker than after a general anaesthetic. It also means that you are awake when your baby is born and your partner may be able to join you in the operating theatre so you can share in the birth together (he is usually asked to sit near your head so he can talk to you, and will be unlikely to be able to see much of the actual surgery). The operation is very quick and your baby is born only minutes after starting the procedure, but stitching you up afterwards takes a while longer. You will probably be in the operating theatre for about half an hour to an hour but you or your partner can usually hold your baby if he is well and has no breathing problems. A midwife will take over your care after the Caesarean and once you have recovered from the immediate effects, you will be transferred to the post-natal ward with your baby (unless he needs to be admitted to the neonatal intensive care unit).

Caesarean section is not without its risks, although the current high rate (30 per cent in the UK, almost 50 per cent in Japan and the USA) means that complications caused by medical staff are negligible because they are so experienced at performing them! Some of the possible complications include prolonged wound or internal bleeding, blood pressure changes, infection in your wound, bladder or chest and difficulty passing urine or stools afterwards, although most of these are usually temporary. More serious complications such as blood clots in your legs or lungs, or rupture of the scar are rare. Your baby is at a very slight risk of distress, but this can usually be relieved quickly by giving him oxygen and will be dependent on whether the Caesarean was planned or an emergency situation.

Recovery from a Caesarean takes much longer than most mothers realize, probably the best part of a year, as you have not only had a baby, but also a major abdominal operation, like having your appendix out, at the same time. It used to be said that 'once a Caesarean, always a Caesarean' as a scar on your uterus from a previous Caesarean is a weak spot, which can become stressed during a subsequent labour. It is possible to have a normal vaginal birth after a Caesarean (VBAC), although it will depend on the reasons for the previous surgery and the progress of a subsequent pregnancy and labour. Many doctors are reluctant to let you try for a normal birth after a previous Caesarean, but most independent midwives in the UK will be happy to care for you in the next pregnancy, usually on condition that you agree to compromise by going into hospital, in the event of problems occurring in labour.

'I couldn't believe how long it took me to recover from my Caesarean. Obviously it was quite painful at first but I was really surprised at how difficult I found some things for several months afterwards – things like reversing the car into a tight parking space would pull at my tummy muscles, and I couldn't put all the washing on the line in one go because the stretching hurt my back where I'd had the epidural.'

Val, 33, mother to Laura, now aged 13 months

NATURAL REMEDIES TO SUPPORT YOU IF YOU NEED A CAESAREAN

Technique	How to use
Acupressure	• Travel sickness wrist bands are very effective for sickness after operations. • Place the button over the point three fingers up from the wrist crease on your inner arm (see also Chapter 5).
Aromatherapy/ massage	• Ask your partner to massage you before a Caesarean – it is relaxing for both of you. • Safe oils include orange and mandarin (uplifting), ylang ylang, frankincense and lavender (relaxing): four drops in 5 ml of base oil. • Aromatherapy oils cannot be used in the operating theatre as they may interact with anaesthetic gases.

Technique	How to use
	• After a Caesarean, add lavender and tea tree oil to bath water for relaxation, pain relief and to prevent infection.
Bach flower remedies	• Rescue Remedy, four drops neat on your tongue just before a Caesarean may ease anxiety and panic; your partner can use it too! • Rescue Remedy is safe, even though you cannot have anything else to eat or drink and will not interfere with prescribed drugs. • If an emergency Caesarean becomes necessary, try mimulus or rock rose for fear plus Star of Bethlehem to combat shock. • Walnut helps you adapt to change afterwards, olive is good for tiredness or oak if you are exhausted. • If you feel disappointed about having a Caesarean, try gentian and willow.
Herbal medicines	• *Stop all herbal medicines at least two weeks before a planned Caesarean section.* • Tell your anaesthetist if you have an emergency Caesarean and have been taking any herbal remedies, especially ginger. • *Do not* take raspberry leaf in pregnancy if you are to have a planned Caesarean. • Calendula or chamomile cream can be gently applied around the wound to aid healing after a Caesarean.

(Contd)

Technique	How to use
	• Although St John's wort (*hypericum perforatum*) is well known as a wound healing herbal remedy, it should not be taken orally if you are breastfeeding – although the homeopathic version is safe.
Homeopathic remedies	• Arnica combats shock, trauma and bruising and hypericum aids healing – start as soon after a Caesarean as possible. • Take one tablet each of arnica 30C and hypericum 30C every hour on the first day; every two hours on day two; every three hours on day three, then stop. • Arnica cream is available but do not apply it directly to the wound.
Relaxation exercises	• Immediately before your Caesarean, try deep breathing exercises to keep you calm, and afterwards to prevent chest infection. • Gentle ankle circling promotes good circulation in your legs. • Do not forget your pelvic floor exercises – even after a Caesarean, your muscles have been relaxed by pregnancy hormones.

10 THINGS TO REMEMBER

1 Progress in labour is dependent on the interaction between your baby, your bony pelvis and the power of your uterine contractions.

2 Signs that you may be getting ready to go into labour include: a 'nesting' instinct when you rush around cleaning the house, feeling emotionally more ready to face labour, a slight reduction in your baby's movements, an increase in bowel activity and needing to pass urine even more frequently as the baby's head drops into your pelvis.

3 More definite signs that you are in labour include a 'show', regular, painful uterine contractions which increase in length, strength and frequency, and rupture of the bag of membranes surrounding the baby.

4 The first stage of labour involves contractions and dilatation of the cervix until it is 10 cm dilated; this can last between six and 24 hours.

5 The second stage of labour is the birth of the baby; the third stage is the delivery of the placenta (afterbirth).

6 Keeping calm helps to reduce stress hormone levels, which can interfere with labour hormones.

7 Your body is designed to cope with labour and birth – deal with one contraction at a time.

8 There are many self-help techniques which you can use to help you cope with the contractions, but do not be afraid to ask for stronger pain relief if you need it.

9 *If complications arise, ask for explanations from your midwife or doctor, so that you understand what is happening and are in an informed position to make decisions about any necessary treatment.*

10 *Pregnancy lasts from 37 to 43 weeks – so do not rush to start things off too early; if induction of labour is suggested because you are overdue you should ask for a full explanation of why it is necessary.*

Part two: happy birthday!

We have explored some of the issues to prepare for the birth of your baby and looked at ways in which you may be able to help yourself, both in working towards as normal a birth as possible and, if necessary, easing the difficulties that come with some of the common problems related to childbirth. If you can remain as positive as possible, mentally, spiritually and physically, you will have a far greater chance that everything will remain normal. In the event that the labour and your baby's birth are not quite what you expected or wished for, you can still focus on the positive aspects of the event so that you may avoid or reduce any sense of disappointment you may experience. For most readers, it is hoped that the day of your baby's birth is one to remember with joy, a sense of achievement, with wonder at what has happened – and with love, for your baby, for your partner and for yourself.

Top tip
Remember: Think positive!

Part three

Positive post-natal

10

Emotions and feelings

In this chapter you will learn:
- *how to cope with your emotions and feelings in the early post-natal period*
- *how to adapt to life with a new baby*
- *how to cope if things were not as you expected.*

This third section focuses on the early days after the delivery and is mostly directed towards helping you to meet your own needs, rather than exploring how to care for your baby, as there are many other excellent books and websites available to help you with this (see Taking it further). The first month with your new baby can be overwhelmingly confusing and full of anxiety, and this section, as with the sections on pregnancy and labour, is designed to help you feel more in control of your situation. It is possible that you may first read this section while you are still pregnant, so some of the content is geared towards helping you to make decisions in advance, although it is also intended to help you make those decisions at any time.

Finally meeting and greeting your new baby is, for most mothers and fathers, the most exciting, wonderful, fascinating, awe-inspiring and uplifting feeling you may ever experience. You will marvel at the miracle of birth and feel proud that you have achieved something so special. You will want to spend hours simply looking at your baby, wondering about his future and what he will become, and may be moved to tears with the absolute joy of it all. You will explore every millimetre of his tiny body and enjoy the sensations when he curls his tiny hand around your finger. You will soak up the wonderful aroma of your baby's skin and revel in the feel of him against your shoulder or on your breast. You will feel deliriously happy, despite being more tired than you ever thought possible.

You will also, no doubt, be overwhelmed by the immense sense of responsibility for this tiny human being and may panic about how you are going to manage. You may worry about how and when to feed him, whether he is wrapped up warmly enough or too much, his varying crying patterns and what they mean, and may react to every new little thing that he does, wondering if he is becoming ill or not. As a parent, every age of your child will bring new worries and anxieties, but all of these feelings and emotions are perfectly normal, and in time you will come to learn how to cope with them. That does not mean the concerns will disappear, just that you will know how to put them in perspective so that they do not take over your entire enjoyment of being a parent.

Top tip
Remember: you do not have to be a 'perfect' parent – you just have to be 'good enough'. It is normal to make some mistakes – but learn from them and think about how to do things differently next time.

Whatever your friends and family have said about the joys and worries of having a new baby, it will still be a complete shock – nothing prepares you for this momentous change in your life. Initially, you are likely to feel completely bemused and confused by what has happened to you. This feeling should soon pass, as it is partly due to your hormones (again!), which are shifting about as they readjust after the birth, so it is normal to feel physically and emotionally stressed in the first few weeks after delivery. You may also still be physically uncomfortable, especially if you suffer 'after pains', have stitches, are getting to grips with breastfeeding or have had a Caesarean section (see Chapter 13).

You may feel particularly insecure, lacking in confidence and unsure about what to do if you have previously had a job or high-powered career that required you to juggle numerous balls while standing on your head, something which you were able to do almost without thinking about it. Even if you did not previously work in paid employment, even if you have already had children, and even if you are fortunate enough to be able to pay for extra help with childcare or domestic duties, you will still feel the same, to a greater or lesser degree. It may take you a few weeks to settle into your routine and learn how to cope with your new responsibilities.

Try not to panic about these feelings – imagine you are starting a new job about which you know nothing – and allow others to show you the ropes. Think about the ways in which you might approach your new job and use the same strategies to cope with new motherhood. Remember, too, that if you were changing to a completely new job, you would normally have a period of training to prepare you, and then go through a phase of transition as you become more familiar with your responsibilities. Why assume that this new role of motherhood is any different, just because it is a normal life event, especially as, with smaller families these days, many of us have little or no previous experience of babies?

How to approach your new role as a mother

Tips for starting a new job	Tips for starting your new role as a mother
• Take time off before you start your new job to give yourself time to rest and prepare.	• Try to start your maternity leave as early as finances will allow to give yourself time to rest and to prepare for labour and your new baby. *(Contd)*

Tips for starting a new job	Tips for starting your new role as a mother
• Do some research to find out about your role and responsibilities and what will be expected of you.	• Read books, search the Internet, join antenatal classes; start thinking about childminders and what to do if you return to work.
• Introduce yourself to the people you will be working with, get to know them and their ways of working; ask questions to find out as much as possible.	• Get to know your baby so you understand him and his behaviour; seek out other expectant and new mothers; get to know your midwife, health visitor and doctor; ask questions to find out as much as possible.
• Plan what you are going to wear, your route to your new place of work and how long it will take you.	• Get organized! Stock the freezer with prepared meals; treat yourself to a new easy-to-manage hairstyle; pack your labour bag and arrange things for when you return home with your new baby; plan your route to the hospital or birth centre.
• Work out what the priorities of the job are likely to be.	• Make lists of priorities – and identify things that are not such a priority (such as housework).
• Be realistic about what you can achieve and do not try to change everything at once.	• Be realistic about what you can achieve each day; do not try to take on too much in one go.

Tips for starting a new job	Tips for starting your new role as a mother
• It takes time to learn a new job; it is normal to make a few mistakes.	• Do not feel that you have to know everything straight away; it is normal to make some mistakes and parenting is a *lifelong* learning experience.
• Have lunch with different people in the organization to get to know them.	• Make dates to meet up with friends, both those with children and those without.
• When the going gets tough, remember that your employer appointed you above all the other candidates.	• When the going gets tough, remember that your baby will love you whatever you do.
• Take care of yourself – get plenty of rest, exercise and sleep, eat well and take time out for yourself.	• Take care of yourself – get plenty of rest, exercise and sleep, eat well and take time out for yourself.
• Celebrate your achievements and successes; enjoy the perks of the job and reward yourself for a job well done.	• Enjoy your baby and your new role as a mother; plan little treats for yourself to look forward to and to remind you that you are a great mother.
• Keep a positive attitude and a positive mind.	• Keep a positive attitude and a positive mind.

There are many normal emotional upheavals in the first week or two after delivery, which can take you by surprise, even if you are expecting them. Post-natal 'blues' occur in about 80 per cent of new mothers and are caused by hormonal mood changes due to the sudden decline in labour hormones and the upsurge in post-natal hormones, especially those required for lactation (which 'kick in' even if you are not breastfeeding). They commonly occur around the third, fourth or fifth day after the birth and seem to hit you suddenly, making you burst into tears for no apparent reason, feel irritable, sad, anxious, exhausted and nervous, and sometimes giving you a sense of anti-climax now that your baby is finally here. These feelings are completely normal and to be expected, require no medical treatment and usually only last for a few days.

Insight

Post-natal 'blues' are normal and are caused by the shifting hormone levels as your body readjusts back to being non-pregnant. Post-natal depression is more serious and often occurs after a few weeks and can last for weeks or months. Post-natal psychosis (mania) is a serious but less common disorder, again caused by changing hormone levels, but most often occurring in women with a personal or family history of mental illness. They are all, however, treatable, if diagnosed early.

Your partner can help at this time by being as supportive and loving as possible, understanding that your tearfulness and irritability should not be confused with post-natal depression. Prepare your partner during pregnancy for the fact that the 'blues' are extremely common and extremely normal. Warn him that it is like premenstrual tension, if you experienced this before pregnancy. Ask him to let you talk about how you feel without the need to resolve anything – there is, in any case, little that can be done to treat the 'blues', although you can take steps to cope with them. Ask him to take on some of the usual household chores for a while until you *feel* more organized and better able to cope, or get help if it is available and/or you can afford it, for example, doing shopping online or sending ironing out to the dry cleaner's.

'At first it would take me nearly all day to get myself washed and dressed because there always seemed so many other things to do to look after Lizzie. One day a parcel arrived at 3 o'clock in the afternoon and I was still in my dressing gown, with my hair uncombed and no make-up on my face. Lizzie was screaming for a feed, the phone was ringing and there was rubbish just inside the front door, waiting to be put in the bin. I don't know what the postman thought of me because he was used to seeing me leave at 7 o'clock wearing my executive suit!'

Susie, 40, stockbroker and mother to Lizzie, aged 6 months

Your partner can also experience a form of 'post-natal blues', perhaps because he has worries about finances, his ability to be a good father or his responsibilities, which can be similar to the feelings which you have at this time. Men traditionally and culturally do not always talk about their feelings, which can make the situation worse, so it is important that he chats to a male friend or family member or that he feels able to inform his doctor or talk to your health visitor about it if it continues.

Although post-natal 'blues' are normal, your partner and family can take note if they seem to persist beyond the first week, when they may also begin to note other signs that suggest you have not yet recovered. Post-natal depression is a more serious condition that can occur any time up to two years after your baby's birth, and although the textbooks will tell you that it affects only about ten per cent of mothers, in reality it is probably many more, as some mild depression goes unnoticed or unreported. If, after a few weeks, you feel miserable all the time, are constantly crying or irritable, exhausted, unable to cope, guilty and resentful of your baby, unable to sleep, have either no appetite or are 'comfort eating', have lost your zest for living, your sex drive and your sense of humour and are unable to enjoy yourself, you may be developing post-natal depression and should consult your health visitor or doctor.

Post-natal depression is more likely to occur if you have had depression before, either prior to or during pregnancy or following the birth of another child, although this is not inevitable. It may also be more likely to develop if there is a family member who has suffered depression, or if your mother died before you became pregnant. It can also develop when your personal, social and domestic circumstances are difficult, such as if you have no support or are the victim of domestic violence, if you have housing or financial worries, or if you or your baby is unwell. Medical treatment primarily consists of counselling and psychotherapy and occasionally the use of medications (see Taking it further).

If your baby's birth did not go according to plan

You and your partner may feel particularly upset and disappointed if your baby's birth was not as you had expected it to be. This may be because developments during labour may have meant that your baby needed to be born by forceps or Caesarean, that you were transferred from home to hospital for the birth, that you required labour to be induced or accelerated, or because you were treated in a way which left you both feeling out of control and powerless, or with loss of dignity and support. It is important to discuss your labour and the birth of your baby with the professional who was responsible for your care at the time. This will give you the opportunity to express your feelings and to seek explanations for anything that you did not understand. If you have specific worries or questions, make an appointment for a formal meeting with the midwife, obstetrician or maternity services manager. Make sure that your community midwife, health visitor and family doctor are aware of how you feel and take every opportunity available to discuss it with them further. They may refer you for more specialized counselling or de-briefing services if it is appropriate. If these feelings are left unresolved, it can trigger post-natal depression and even develop into a form of post-traumatic stress disorder (PTSD) in which you experience 'flashbacks', nightmares and behavioural changes. This is now recognized as a rare but serious complication following childbirth, for which treatment is available. If it is not treated, PTSD can become a chronic problem that affects you, your partner and your family, and may lead you to avoid subsequent pregnancies (see Taking it further).

Insight

Birth de-briefing should be offered by the midwife who cared for you during labour. If it is not offered, ask to speak to one of the midwives while you are still in contact with them. If necessary, write and ask for an appointment with the Head of Midwifery.

10 THINGS TO REMEMBER

1 *You do not have to be a 'perfect' parent – mistakes are normal.*

2 *DO NOT PANIC! Take your time and use your common sense – and you will do the 'right thing'.*

3 *Try to get as organized as possible, preferably before your baby is born.*

4 *Post-natal 'blues' are normal but if you feel excessively low, or can't stop crying, or if your partner notices that you seem depressed, consult your midwife, doctor or health visitor.*

5 *Try to talk to your midwife about your baby's birth, especially if there were complications, so that you understand what happened and can be prepared for any future pregnancy. If necessary ask for an appointment with your obstetric consultant.*

6 *Try to see friends, or meet other new mothers so that you do not feel isolated with your new baby, especially if you are not returning to work.*

7 *Feeling overwhelmed is normal – but just take each day as it comes.*

8 *Eat well and get adequate rest, sleep and exercise.*

9 *Share any concerns with your partner, a friend or a trusted professional.*

10 *ENJOY your baby – he is not tiny for long!*

11

Sex and relationships

In this chapter you will learn:
- *how a new baby can affect your family relationships*
- *when to resume sex*
- *about suggested methods of contraception.*

Family dynamics

The arrival of a new baby dramatically changes the dynamics within the family. In years gone by, families lived in close-knit communities and everyone helped everyone else. Grandparents often lived nearby and were available to help with childcare on the odd occasion that the parents were occupied elsewhere. Nowadays, of course, many women work in full-time employment, at least until the birth of their first baby, but they often live some distance away from other family members, and some new parents have very little readily available, local help.

Grandparents can be a help or a hindrance, depending on how far away you live from them, your relationship with them prior to and during your pregnancy and how much help they want to give and you wish to accept. If your mother or mother-in-law offers advice only when you ask for it, you will welcome her involvement, and older women have much to offer in the way of personal life experiences. They can also be a little more objective than you at this stage, not least because they do not have hugely fluctuating hormone levels with which to contend. However, if she is constantly critical of your efforts, perhaps comparing you to herself, your sister or sister-in-law, this can cause friction, which can build up a sense of resentment (on both sides) and adversely affect your enjoyment of the early days with your baby. She may find it difficult to accept that many theories about childcare and raising children have changed since she was a new mother, such as the use of 'on demand breastfeeding', involvement of your partner in caring for your baby or the fact that you want to go back to work fairly soon after the birth. It can be hard to accept unwanted advice with good grace but it may reduce tensions if you can do this. Try telling her that your ideas are based on good sources of information from books/the Internet/antenatal classes, thank her for her thoughts and put them to one side for later consideration. Remember that this is your baby and you are entitled to do things your own way, but be careful not to over-react to her suggestions simply because you are feeling unsure.

Siblings

Your other children may respond to the arrival of your new baby in a variety of different ways. Small children are often disillusioned that the baby is not yet ready to play with them, and may even be disappointed about the baby's sex, depending on their original wishes. Some parents give siblings a gift 'from the baby' but it is wise to keep this small, to avoid the potential impression of offering an apology for bringing home an 'interloper'. Give your child as much time as you can and involve her in helping you to look after the new arrival. Even a toddler can hand you a nappy or gently stroke your new baby's face to try to stop him crying. Take some photographs of your child sitting on the sofa and holding your baby so that she feels important; perhaps she could take the photograph to nursery school to show everyone. If you are breastfeeding your baby, let your child sit with you and try to put your other arm round her so that she does not feel left out. With toddlers and very young children, there can be signs of regression to infancy such as wanting to go on your breast again (usually this is just a request for attention and she will probably not try it more than a couple of times), or starting to wet the bed or eating with a baby spoon. Sibling rivalry can be exhibited with anger, tears, frustration and misbehaviour or, occasionally, with exaggeratedly good behaviour and expressions of undying love for the new arrival. These should not normally be a problem and usually settle down fairly quickly but if you are worried, contact your health visitor or family doctor. Set a few simple boundaries that your child can understand, such as not picking the baby up when you are not there and not touching him with toys (exuberance can mean that 'touch' is rather more forceful than they intended). Be gentle but firm and consistent with your rules and discipline so that she understands that your baby is here to stay.

Insight

If your other children start behaving badly, try not to reprimand them too much, or do so in such as way that they will not come to resent the new baby. Positive 'carrots' are better than negative 'sticks'!

Pets and the new baby

Your pet is also likely to react to your new baby, especially if he has been the 'baby' of the family and accustomed to your undivided attention (see Chapter 3 on suggestions for preparing your cat or dog during pregnancy). In many respects, you have to treat your pet as if he were another child in order to avoid any jealousy. It is rare for dogs not to adjust to a new arrival, although cats can take rather longer and may spend more time outside than previously. Be firm with your pet but try to differentiate simple inquisitiveness from determined attempts to harm your baby. It is important at this early stage to set and adhere to ground rules, not only to avoid problems of a jealous pet, but also to reduce the risk of your baby developing allergic reactions to animal hair. Always wash your hands after handling or playing with your pet before touching your baby, and ensure that your cat or dog is regularly treated for infections and infestations such as fleas, worms and other diseases that could be transmitted to your baby. If you have your baby in hospital or in a birthing centre, it may help to speed up a dog's acceptance if your partner brings home something with your baby's 'smell' on it, such as a worn (unsoiled) item of clothing or a small blanket which has been in the cot, so that when you and your baby return home your dog will be familiar with the smell. On your arrival back home, spend some time with your pet to assure him that he is still important to you. Insist that dogs and cats stay out of the baby's room/cot unless you are there (beware of leaving windows open in ground floor rooms to which your cat may have access). It is a myth that cats will consciously smother a baby but they do seem to like the warmth of the cot and may decide to curl up near your baby's face if left unattended. A cat may become aggravated by the sound of your baby's crying and try to explore the source by jumping onto the cot/pram if he can. Some cats seem to dislike the smell of breast milk so he may ignore you while you are lactating; ensure that he is not in the room while you are breastfeeding.

'Before I had Adam, you could set your clock by Mogsie, our 14-year-old cat: she always used to come in for supper at 5 o'clock. After Adam was born, it was a miracle some days if she came in at all, at least until my husband came home.'

Denise, mother to Adam, 18

Family planning

You may have already made some decisions about whether and when to have more children after this baby, or it may be something you need to consider now. Your decisions may be based on how many children you have already, how this pregnancy and birth progressed, finances, housing, jobs and your personal, family and cultural perspectives and philosophy. How much time you wish to leave between pregnancies is a very personal decision, and there is no 'right' answer, although bear in mind that your body physically takes about a year to recover fully from each pregnancy and birth.

Many midwives and obstetricians advise waiting about six to eight weeks before resuming sex, so that you will have had your post-natal follow-up appointment, but there is some rationale for trying sex before this as it can highlight physical problems such as unhealed vaginal tears or stitches which have not dissolved but which can be diagnosed during your medical examination and treated quickly. Again, the decision about when to restart sex is very individual and may depend on how much blood loss you have, whether you have had stitches or a Caesarean section and your health and that of your baby. You may not immediately feel physically or emotionally ready for sex, especially as you may be very tired and engrossed in your new baby, but try not to ignore your partner's needs too.

Finding time to restart sex can be quite difficult and you may need to be flexible and make changes from your old routine. Do not assume you will only have sex when you go to bed at night – you may both be so tired that all you want to do is to fall asleep! Consider planning to have sex in the afternoon when your baby is sleeping during the day. Ask friends to look after your baby for a few hours, while you cook a nice meal, take a shower together or give each other a massage to get you in the mood. At first it may be necessary to arrange a date and time for sex, but bear in mind that you may not feel like it when you eventually get together. If that is the case, just enjoy being with each other.

Making a bedtime routine is vital as your baby gets older and is something you may like to consider even from the early months. One of the most common reasons for sexual dissatisfaction among parents – and for the ultimate breakdown in some relationships – is that children are permitted to stay up all evening, preventing the parents from having undisturbed 'adult' time, not necessarily sexual, but simply being able to talk and behave as adults. Make a pact with your partner *now* to be very firm about bedtimes so that the evening can be *your* time. If you start this habit early, your children will conform without any difficulties, will be more disciplined and better behaved, better humoured, more rested, more alert, more sociable and better able to learn well at school than if you allow too much freedom over bedtimes.

The first occasion on which you decide to have sex is likely to be a little uncomfortable, because your vagina can be quite dry in the early weeks after giving birth. You may feel rather anxious about it, but persevere and do not force the issue. A vaginal lubricant can be useful, but use a water soluble one if you are using condoms for contraception, and avoid those with colourings, flavourings or fragrances as these can cause irritation in the early weeks after delivery. If you cannot manage full penetrative sex for a while, express your love for one another in other ways: you could, for example, try mutual masturbation or indulge in oral sex. Be aware that breast and nipple stimulation will trigger your 'let down' reflex and you are likely to leak some milk, even if you are not breastfeeding. You may have to choose a sexual position that does not put pressure on any parts of your body that still feel painful or uncomfortable, for example, your abdomen if you have had a Caesarean section.

Insight

If you have had an episiotomy you may wish to wait until the stitches have dissolved before trying sex. However, occasionally a stitch is left inside and this can come out during sex – or cause discomfort during penetration. Do not panic, but let you midwife, health visitor or doctor know – they may examine you to check that everything is progressing normally.

CASE STUDY

'The first time we tried it after Jules's birth was after we'd been out for a meal. We'd left him with a friend who had a girl of the same age, but while we were in the restaurant all we could talk about was if Jules was OK without us, so we went back to collect him after only an hour and a half. We went home and had a glass of wine and decided to try sex, but I was so tired and stressed out that it was a complete failure. Laurie was very good about it and said it didn't matter, and we just went to sleep holding each other.'

Beccy, 24, mother to Jules and partner of Laurie, 26

Contraception

Whatever your decisions about family spacing and when to resume sex, it is important to think about the best method of contraception for you both. The following tables explain the main methods of contraception available, with advantages and disadvantages, to help you to make decisions that suit you both.

CONDOM – MALE

How it works	Positive aspects
• acts as barrier between penis and vagina • usually used with spermicidal gels for extra effectiveness.	• 98 per cent effective if used correctly • cheap, easily available • does not need medical check • reduces risk of sexually transmitted infections.
Possible problems	Reasons to avoid it
• may be uncomfortable in early post-natal period (dryness) • may split if put on roughly • oil-based lubricants will cause tears in latex condoms • interferes with spontaneity • may cause allergy if latex • should never be re-used.	• if you have a latex allergy (in which case, ensure you buy latex-free condoms).

CONDOM – FEMALE

How it works	Positive aspects
• insert into vagina before sex • lines whole vaginal cavity.	• possibly 95 per cent effective • designed primarily to prevent sexually transmitted infections.

Possible problems	Reasons to avoid it
• can be painful with stitches • interferes with spontaneity • easy to insert penis between condom and vaginal wall by mistake.	• unreliable in early post-natal period due to stretching of vaginal wall – wait 6–8 weeks • if you want more effectiveness.

CAP – INCLUDING DIAPHRAGM

How it works	Positive aspects
• diaphragm fits in top of vagina as barrier • cervical cap fits onto outer cervix • fitted at family planning clinic • used with spermicidal gel • best inserted routinely at night.	• 92–96 per cent effective • suitable for older mothers • suitable when Pill/coil are not • cheap, easy to use and readily available.

Possible problems	Reasons to avoid it
• may cause allergy • may cause cystitis • incorrect fit if you lose or gain more than 3 kg in weight.	• if you have had toxic shock syndrome.

Insight

It is unlikely that your cap or diaphragm which you used before pregnancy will fit securely enough after giving birth. You will need to get it checked (to make sure it is safe) and you may have to wait a few weeks until after your post-natal appointment to ensure that your body has returned to normal before using this method, so it may be necessary to use an alternative for the first few weeks.

NATURAL FAMILY PLANNING

(including rhythm method and commercial aids such as Persona™)

How it works	Positive aspects
• based on awareness of own body and menstrual cycle to find fertile periods	• you are totally in control
	• no side effects of hormones
• sex is avoided during fertile periods	• no medical check needed
	• may help when planning next pregnancy.
• calendar method	
• temperature method	
• mucus method	
• Persona™ – detects changing urine hormone levels for 'safe' phase.	

Possible problems	Reasons to avoid it
• not reliable contraceptive	• if you want guaranteed effective contraception
• need 3–4 months of regular menstrual cycles before start	• if you want sex during fertile phases
• needs motivation from both partners	• if you do not have time to take your temperature/test urine every morning.
• mucus examination difficult after sex	
• Persona™ unreliable if on certain medications.	

Sometimes after childbirth your menstrual cycle changes radically, so it would not be wise to rely on natural family planning for several months until you have charted your 'new' menstrual cycle and are sure about when you ovulate. Obviously you cannot use this method while breastfeeding as your hormones are different at this time.

INTRAUTERINE CONTRACEPTIVE DEVICE (COIL)

How it works	Positive aspects
• T-shaped device of plastic or silver fitted inside uterus • attached to two threads – hang down inside top of Vagina • check threads regularly • interferes with lining of uterus and mucus to prevent pregnancy.	• 98 per cent effective • suitable 6–8 weeks after childbirth • you can forget about it – lasts between five and eight years • can be used as emergency contraception.
Possible problems	Reasons to avoid it
• can be uncomfortable to fit • can cause heavy periods • can irritate Chlamydia infection • may come out • can cause infection • may cause ectopic pregnancy • can perforate uterus (rare).	• if you have active Chlamydia • previous ectopic pregnancy • if you suffer heavy periods (tend to get better after childbirth) • need to wait 6–8 weeks after delivery • may not be suitable if you have not had a baby – insertion of the coil can be very painful if the cervix (neck of the uterus) has not been stretched by childbirth and is still tightly closed.

INTRAUTERINE SYSTEM (MIRENA™ COIL)

How it works	Positive aspects
• similar shape to coil but contains hormones • steady release of hormones • thickens cervical mucus • thins lining of uterus • may suppress ovulation.	• 99 per cent effective • less painful and lighter periods • does not interfere with sex • lasts for five years.

Possible problems	Reasons to avoid it
• can take a few months to take effect • initially irregular periods • breast tenderness • spots, acne • headaches • cysts on your ovaries • may fall out • may perforate uterus (rare).	• unexplained vaginal bleeding • pelvic/uterine infections • abnormal shaped uterus • heart conditions (valves).

CONTRACEPTIVE INJECTION

How it works	Positive aspects
• injection into buttock muscle • stops ovulation, thickens mucus, thins lining of uterus • Depo Provera™ lasts 12 weeks – progesterone • Noristerat™ lasts eight weeks – progesterone • Lunelle™ (new) combined oestrogen/progesterone.	• 99 per cent effective • does not interfere with sex • suitable when breastfeeding • may protect against cancer of uterus.

(Contd)

Possible problems	Reasons to avoid it
• increased risk of breast cancer • heavy, prolonged periods • infrequent/absent periods • headache, nausea • abdominal pain • weight gain • dizziness, weakness • may affect other medications • may affect future fertility.	• if you want to get pregnant again fairly quickly • family history of breast cancer • if you are overweight • previous infertility problems • suffer from migraines • liver disease • history of thrombosis (clots) • family history of osteoporosis.

CONTRACEPTIVE IMPLANTS

How it works	Positive aspects
• hormone implant under skin in upper arm • steady flow of hormones released into bloodstream • stops ovulation.	• 99–100 per cent effective • does not interfere with breastfeeding • can be inserted 3–4 weeks after childbirth • can be removed if problems occur • lasts for three years.

Possible problems	Reasons to avoid it
• can affect sex drive • headaches, nausea • spots, acne • weight gain • breast tenderness • dizziness, fainting • depression • can move from site of insertion.	• unexplained vaginal bleeding • history of pregnancy itching • history of thrombosis • have ovarian cysts • if you are very overweight • taking drugs for epilepsy • taking drugs for tuberculosis • previous cancers.

CONTRACEPTIVE PATCH

How it works	Positive aspects
• new – combined hormones in patch attached to skin • similar to Pill but via skin • each patch lasts one week • use for three weeks, rest for one week.	• 99 per cent effective if used correctly • does not cause nausea as with Pill • unaffected by diarrhoea as with Pill.

Possible problems	Reasons to avoid it
• breast tenderness • nausea, headache, migraine • spots, acne • vaginal 'spotting' • flu-like symptoms (temporary) • patch may come off • skin irritation where attached • does not reduce period pain.	• if you are overweight • if you are forgetful • severe recurrent migraines • history of thrombosis.

PROGESTERONE–ONLY CONTRACEPTIVE PILL (MINI PILL)

How it works	Positive aspects
• thickens mucus around uterus/cervix – stops sperm entering • thins lining of uterus so less receptive to fertilized eggs • partially stops you ovulating.	• 98 per cent effective • suitable when breastfeeding • suitable for diabetics, high blood pressure, smokers, older women • suitable when oestrogen is not.

(Contd)

Possible problems	Reasons to avoid it
• must be taken same time each day • if more than three hours late – use alternative till next period • irregular/no periods • breast tenderness • nausea, headaches • skin discolouration/spots • ectopic pregnancy possible.	• if you forget to take tablets • you work irregular hours • if you are overweight • unexplained vaginal bleeding • previous ectopic pregnancy • very high cholesterol • artery disease • history of breast cancer.

COMBINED CONTRACEPTIVE PILL (ORAL)

How it works	Positive aspects
• oestrogen and progesterone • prevents ovulation • take for 21 days, rest for seven • alternatively, take every day, with seven 'dummy' tablets • withdrawal bleed in rest week mimics a period.	• almost 100 per cent effective • stops painful periods • periods shorter and lighter • reduces risk of anaemia • may improve acne • reduced risk of ovary, uterus, bowel cancer.

Possible problems	Reasons to avoid it
• headaches, migraine, nausea • breast tenderness, weight gain • 'spotting' between periods • increased blood pressure • varicose veins • ineffective with diarrhoea or with certain antibiotics • thrombosis, heart attack (rare) • increased risk of breast, cervical, liver cancer.	• if you are breastfeeding • if you are a smoker • high blood pressure • family history of thrombosis • if you are overweight, • high cholesterol • varicose or inflamed veins • diabetic • history of breast cancer • aged 35 or over.

STERILIZATION – FEMALE

How it works	Positive aspects
• blocking or cutting and tying of fallopian tubes • usually done via tiny incision near your 'belly button'.	• 100 per cent effective • takes effect immediately.

Possible problems	Reasons to avoid it
• permanent • difficult if you are overweight • difficult to reverse • infections, trauma from surgery • small risk of ectopic pregnancy.	• if you want more children • if you have fibroids or ovarian cysts • if you have a prolapsed uterus • if you have pelvic inflammatory disease.

STERILIZATION – MALE (VASECTOMY)

How it works	Positive aspects
• operation to cut the tubes carrying sperm from testicles • done under local anaesthetic.	• almost 100 per cent effective; permanent • does not interfere with sex • quick, easy, fairly painless • safer than female sterilization.

Possible problems	Reasons to avoid it
• may reduce sex drive • not easily reversible • sperm still produced up to six months • may raise blood pressure • may increase risk of prostate cancer.	• if you want more children • if you have not yet had children.

Insight

If you choose for either you or your partner to be sterilized you must be certain that this is what you want. Although there have been reversals of sterilization, you should consider these to be permanent life choices.

10 THINGS TO REMEMBER

1 *A new baby in the family affects everyone – you, your partner, your children, your parents, even your pets.*

2 *You started as a couple, so take time to be together as a couple, occasionally leaving your baby with someone else for an hour or two.*

3 *If you have other children, consider ways of introducing the new arrival to them so that they do not feel 'left out' of all the excitement.*

4 *Resuming sex can be difficult – but try it before your six-week post-natal appointment so that any physical problems as a consequence of the birth, e.g. stitiches which have not dissolved, can be treated.*

5 *Don't rush things, stay calm and if sex is too uncomfortable, just cuddle and be with each other.*

6 *Develop a routine for your baby so that as he grows up he recognizes when it is bedtime, leaving you and your partner to have the evening to yourselves.*

7 *Do NOT forget contraception!*

8 *Talk to your midwife, health visitor, doctor or practice nurse, or visit a family planning clinic to decide which method of contraception is best for you.*

9 *Some types of contraception may be best avoided for a few weeks until your body has readjusted after the birth, e.g. condom, intrauterine coil.*

10 *It takes your body, especially your skeleton, a year to recover from pregnancy, so you may prefer to wait a while before trying for another baby, but this is a very personal decision.*

12

....

Work, rest and play

In this chapter you will learn:
- *how to get organized at home and work*
- *how to deal with visitors*
- *ways to ensure adequate rest and sleep*
- *how to cope with your crying baby*
- *how to get some 'time out' for you and your partner*
- *about the issues surrounding the decision to return to work.*

The sooner you can get your new life with your baby into some semblance of order, the easier it will be. You will feel more in control and have more time and energy to enjoy your baby. This is truly a case of prioritizing, although in the early days it can seem almost impossible to get organized. You may be conscious that you are still in your dressing gown in the middle of the afternoon, have not put on any make-up for four days and are surrounded by piles of washing-up, ironing or clothes to be laundered.

Do not panic! This is normal and it does not matter.
Many midwives and health visitors would be wary of entering the house of a newborn baby to find it spotlessly tidy. This may mean either that the family was focusing on housework rather than getting to know their baby, or that the mother was becoming exhausted and at risk of post-natal depression with all the effort of not only caring for a baby but also doing all the housework. However, there are ways in which you can make things a little

easier so that you can concentrate on organizing your new life in order that you can once again feel in control of things.

Get as organized as you can in advance, i.e. during pregnancy. Make a range of meals to put in the freezer and do as many of the larger household chores as you can manage, such as washing curtains or decorating. Sort out any repairs and stock up on things you may forget, like washing powder and light bulbs. Ensure that you have completed those tasks that crop up annually, for example, the car's MOT, your pet's immunizations, children's dental examinations or renewing household insurances (and if your partner usually takes responsibility for some of these jobs, get him to check them out before your baby is born, as he may also forget later). Prepare a list of all the people you will want to notify about the birth and either make an email group list or write the envelopes if you intend to send birth notification cards by post. If you have the energy in the last few weeks before the birth, 'spring clean' your house from top to bottom, one room at a time, so that you will not have to think about this for some time afterwards. Sort out your clothes for when you have had your baby (but do not expect to be able to get back into your jeans straight away!) and make sure everything is washed, ironed, repaired and put away. Arrange rotas of friends and neighbours to take your other children to school for the first few weeks after the birth, perhaps to have them home after school one afternoon a week, or to walk your dog each morning and evening.

Once you are home with your new baby, make a list of the priorities in your family's life. At this early stage, it is natural that your baby should come first, but you must come next. You owe it to your family to keep well and happy so that their time with you and your new baby can be a positive experience and not one on which they could look back with negative feelings because everyone is stressed, disorganized and irritable. Do not try to do too much – set yourself just one main household task each day, such as putting washing in the machine or going to the laundrette, or ironing, or cooking to stock up the freezer, or shopping. If you find it difficult to do a full weekly shop at the supermarket, walk to your local shops each day and buy only the few things you need for that day. This will have the extra advantages of making you get out in the fresh air with your baby, getting some exercise and meeting people, even if it is only strangers in the shops or the park. Below are some more suggestions for making time for yourself by organizing housework chores.

Ways to reduce housework

▶ *Use baskets or boxes for different items, e.g. one for toys, one for socks, etc. – throw things in and sort them out later.*
▶ *Put a basket at the foot of the staircase to collect anything that needs taking upstairs.*
▶ *Keep a wipe-clean board in the kitchen to note down things you need to do or buy.*
▶ *Put all your household bills in one file or tray; mark payment dates on the kitchen calendar.*
▶ *Use commercial 'ready wipes' for housework – they are more expensive but easier and quicker.*
▶ *Save all your supermarket carrier bags for kitchen rubbish and make one trip daily to the rubbish bin.*
▶ *Tidy up as you go along each day – this is easier than one big weekly clear-up.*
▶ *Involve older children in picking up their own toys, clearing the table, etc. with rewards for good work; make a game of it for them.*
▶ *Keep a bag ready packed – and restocked – with all the things you need for your baby when you go out.*
▶ *Keep two laundry baskets in the bathroom for light and dark laundry to save having to separate them later.*
▶ *Put a load of washing in the machine to wash overnight, then dry in the morning.*
▶ *Put socks and small items in a mesh bag to avoid having to sort them out.*
▶ *Separate out forks, knives, spoons, etc. into separate sections in the dishwasher.*
▶ *Keep a bowl of water ready to soak very heavily caked-on cooking utensils before washing.*

> ▶ *Invest in a slow cooker, vegetable steamer or learn how to cook one-pot meals to reduce washing up.*
> ▶ *When you leave work, ask friends to give you a gift of 'housework tokens' so they can do small chores for you when you need them.*
> ▶ *Cook double amounts of food and freeze half.*
> ▶ *Plan weekly menus and keep the list in the kitchen – this avoids the need to think about what to cook and reduces shopping.*
> ▶ *Keep some supermarket 'ready-prepared' meals in the freezer for emergencies*
> ▶ *Shop online for groceries.*

You may have discussed beforehand what you expect your partner to do – he may be rather reluctant to change nappies, for example. However, 'sharing the chores' does not mean each of you doing 50 per cent of *each* chore, but doing a 50 per cent division of the workload – so, if he is happy doing all the heavy tasks such as cleaning the cars, putting out the rubbish and mowing the lawn, leaving the childcare issues to you, accept gratefully that you are not having to do everything around the house and garden.

Accept any offers of help that are given, whether they are from your partner, mother or mother-in-law, friends or colleagues. If you feel guilty about accepting help, there will always be a time later when you can repay their kindness so be thankful that they have offered. Women are particularly good at helping each other out and many would feel offended if you declined their offers – so learn to say 'yes'. Learn also to ask for help. If a friend is coming to visit, ask her to call in at the shops on her way to bring you something you need but have not had time to buy, or to collect dry cleaning. As they leave, ask family and neighbours to post letters, return children's library books or put the rubbish out in the bins.

Try to find time every day to do something for yourself, so that you attend to your own needs, even if you only have ten minutes. This should not be essential things such as showering, but activities which make you feel better, for example, having a warm relaxing bath instead, or spending ten minutes reading the newspaper or a magazine to remind you that there is life beyond the four walls of your home. How about asking your partner to leave you sleeping for an extra half an hour one morning at the weekend while he looks after your baby? Later, once your routine is established, try to plan a half day each week for *yourself* to do things like go for a swim or to an exercise class, to have your hair done or get your legs waxed, or to catch up on the videos you have recorded when you have been too busy to watch the scheduled television programmes.

Top tip

Try to find time every day to do something you *want* to do, not something you *have* to do.

Develop a routine, based on the priorities you have set yourself. Unless you have had a particularly sleepless night, set your alarm clock to wake you at the same time each morning, and if your baby is still asleep, use this time to sort yourself out, showering, getting dressed and putting on some make-up. This will make you feel more 'human' and you will be ready if any visitors arrive. If you have any time left before your baby demands your attention, you could either start on one of your chores, or simply relax. When your baby sleeps in the daytime, balance your 'free' time with some essential jobs and some relaxation periods. Make sure you go to bed at approximately the same time each night even if you have to get up again soon afterwards to feed your baby.

Dealing with visitors

There will be many family members, friends and neighbours who want to 'drop in' to meet your new baby, but it can be extremely tiring (and noisy) to have a constant stream of people visiting you in the hospital or birth unit, or at home, however well-meaning they are. This can have a 'knock on' effect on the whole family, making everyone irritable and your baby and other children fractious. Towards the end of pregnancy, it is useful to devise a strategy with your partner for dealing with telephone calls and visitors.

In UK maternity units visiting is usually restricted, with only the partner and the mother's own children permitted unrestricted visiting. Visiting hours for others are normally limited and there is usually also a maximum of two visitors allowed at any one time. These restrictions are designed to enable new parents to concentrate on caring for their babies and to rest or sleep when possible. In many maternity units mothers will be in small wards, perhaps with four beds, so it is not just about *your* needs but also those of the other mothers near you. (Imagine how annoyed you would be if you wanted to sleep and the mother in the next bed had four or five visitors with her for several hours). If your own parents, in-laws and friends live locally, you may decide to ask them *not* to visit you in the hospital and to wait until you return home. Obviously it is more difficult if they have travelled from far away and their availability is limited, but perhaps these individuals should be given priority over others who live within easy reach.

Insight

Hospital visitors are also restricted because of the rise in infections such as MRSA and C. difficile, which can both be caught while you are in hospital. Although infection is usually mild, it can be much more serious for people who are susceptible – such as your baby, other small children and even you, during pregnancy and immediately after the birth. Conversely, if children visit who have been in contact with some of the normal childhood illnesses such as mumps or chickenpox, this can also put the babies in the ward at risk, so don't allow your child to visit if this is the case.

Once you are at home it becomes even more difficult to fend off all those who want to meet your new family member. During the first week or two, it is worth considering allocating just *two hours* in each day when you are willing to receive telephone calls – tell your friends and family in advance, and perhaps also remind them via the birth notification cards/emails. Be firm about refusing to answer the telephone outside these hours (leave the answerphone on).You may also wish to arrange just *one* evening or afternoon in the first week when anyone can visit in person, and extend this to two sessions in the second week. Tell them in advance the times you are 'open for visiting' and the times you will want them to leave – and ask your partner to be assertive about this when it comes to asking them to go. It is *not* appropriate for all your visitors to have a cuddle with your baby, which, quite apart from the risk of infection, can upset his routine, making him difficult to settle and leaving you more stressed than you already feel.

While your visitors are in your home, do not feel pressurized to be with them all the time – they have, after all, come to see your new baby – so use the time to catch up on having a rest, a bath or making some essential telephone calls. Do not be afraid to 'use' them – ask each of them to bring something such as an item from your next shopping list (nappies, milk, shampoo) or a dish for supper, or give them a small task to complete while they are with you, such as stacking the dishwasher or doing the washing up, reading a story to your other children or sticking stamps on all those birth notification cards which need sending. If it is warm weather, think about having a barbecue and ask everyone to bring a contribution to the meal so that you do not have to plan, shop, cook and clear up afterwards.

> ### Top tip
> Plan to restrict visitors and telephone calls to a minimum in the first two weeks after your baby's birth, to allow you and your partner time to get to know him, get organized and get some sleep!

> ### Insight
> Do not under-estimate just how tiring and stressful it can be to have a new baby in the house. You are recovering from the birth (and sometimes a major operation as well if you have had a Caesarean), plus you and your partner are both learning how to care for and respond to your baby.

Once you are organized, it is good to get out of the house each day and to meet people, including new mothers, in order to avoid the feeling of isolation that can occur when you are at home on your own. This can be particularly profound if you previously worked in a busy environment, meeting and talking to many different people each day. If you have attended preparation for birth classes during your pregnancy, try to stay in touch with one or two women to whom you relate well so that you can meet up when your babies have been born. There are usually mother and baby/toddler groups in your local area; your health visitor should be able to tell you about them, or contact your local library or nursery for more information. In the UK, Sure Start programmes offer opportunities for you to meet with local mothers who are in similar circumstances to your own. There are also classes and groups designed to help you stimulate your baby from an early age, such as baby massage, swimming or music groups, depending on your family's specific interests, where you will also be able to meet other parents.

Caution: do not make the mistake of assuming that because you have your children in common, you will automatically have things in common with all the adults you meet. If you want to meet like-minded people, ask around your normal social circle during pregnancy to find out about activities that match your particular interests, ideals and philosophies. There is no point in taking your child to baby singing classes if you do not like music or cannot sing, nor would it be easy to join a mother and baby group that regularly ends up in the local burger restaurant if you are vegetarian.

'We didn't develop a wide circle of friends with children until Harriet was 6 months old and went to nursery when I returned to work. However, we met one couple there who seemed very nice and they introduced us to more couples with babies, so now we regularly meet up in one of our houses. We all take a contribution to supper, the men sometimes do a barbecue and all the babies are settled upstairs – and because we're all in the same boat, no one minds if one of them starts crying or needs feeding.'

Fiona, 37, mother of Harriet, now 10 months old

Rest and sleep

Perhaps the single most profound difficulty for new parents is the constant tiredness that they feel, not just from sleepless nights but also due to the stress of new responsibilities, learning new skills and adapting to a new lifestyle. Unfortunately, you will have to get used to having broken sleep at night and using every opportunity in the daytime to catch up. Your newborn baby will sleep for about 20 hours each day so, once your routine is established, you should find time to rest with your feet up at some point. Use the relaxation exercises you learned at your antenatal classes to remind you how to relax both your muscles and your mind. Ask a friend or neighbour whom you trust to look after your baby for a couple of hours while you go to bed.

Ensure you eat well and regularly, especially if you are breastfeeding or have returned to work; have plenty of protein, fresh fruit and vegetables and drink at least two litres of water daily. Carbohydrate foods are best eaten in the evening as they have a sedative effect and make you sleepy. Get some exercise and fresh air every day if you can, as this will help you to sleep better, and try to organize some time for yourself. If you find that you are becoming excessively tired and unable to concentrate or carry on your day-to-day activities, talk to your health visitor, family doctor or local post-natal support group.

Tips for helping you get to sleep

- ▶ *Avoid stimulants before going to bed, e.g. coffee, alcohol, cola, chocolate, cigarettes and activities such as watching TV, sorting out work papers, or those requiring concentration.*
- ▶ *Eat your evening meal before 7 p.m. if possible to allow you to digest the food while you are still awake.*
- ▶ *If you have time, go for a short family stroll for some fresh air after you have eaten.*
- ▶ *Establish a routine at night, going to bed at approximately the same time, doing the same things each evening as you*

prepare for bed, such as having a warm bath, putting a drop of lavender oil on a tissue on your pillow or listening to relaxing music.

▶ *Ensure your bedroom is conducive to sleep by keeping it well ventilated, not too warm, free from television and computer equipment, and only using it for sleeping and sex so that it does not become associated with other, more stimulating activities.*

▶ *Sleep only in your bed – make an effort to get up from the sofa, rocking chair or older child's bed if you find yourself nodding off.*

▶ *Avoid sleeping tablets unless prescribed by your doctor, although occasionally herbal medicines, such as chamomile tea or passiflora capsules, or homeopathic remedies, such as coffea, can be helpful.*

▶ *If you really cannot sleep after you have been in bed for some time do not panic – get up and read a book, have a drink or listen to music for a while and go back to bed later.*

▶ *If you need to get up at a specific time in the morning, to take children to school or to get to work, set your alarm clock, increase the volume so that you will hear it and put it in a place where you will have to get out of bed to turn it off.*

▶ *Prepare everything you need for the next day during the previous evening, e.g. clothes, polished shoes, papers for work, children's lunch boxes, etc. in case you oversleep!*

Coping with your crying baby

One of the main reasons for sleepless nights and irritability is the natural demands of your baby for attention. The only way that a newborn baby can attract your attention is by crying, and most newborns cry for about two to three hours each day, albeit in small phases. Babies cry because they want or need something – food, drink, to be warmer or cooler, to be made more comfortable, such as having their nappy changed, to have a cuddle or to tell you they are in pain or unwell. Occasionally, they will cry because they are so tired that they are unable to get to sleep easily – this is often as a result of being handled by too many people, or may be because you are exposing him to some other excessive stimulation such as noise (e.g. television or radio) or light. It can be useful to keep a 'crying chart' for a while – this will show you exactly how much your baby is actually crying – and may reveal patterns to help you work out the reasons. This can be a good way of showing you that all is well. You may be surprised by what you find!

A 'CRYING CHART'

Time of inset of crying	Minutes since last feed	Minutes since last sleep	Duration of crying (minutes)	What helped him to stop crying ?	Duration of sleeping (minutes)

Learn to recognize your baby's cry and what each different cry means, by experimenting with some of the suggestions opposite. At this early stage, he will not have learned to demand your attention simply for the sake of it, as some older children do, so always attend to him and see if you can find out what he is trying to tell you. If you respond to him in this way, you will soon learn to appreciate his crying and not to see it as a nuisance or irritation. If your baby continues to cry and you are unable to pacify him, do not worry too much. Babies will not be harmed by occasionally being left to cry while you take a break to gather your thoughts together. However, if there are significant changes in his normal crying pattern or if the tone of his cry alters dramatically, do consult your doctor to ensure your baby is not becoming unwell.

'I found it really difficult at first, trying to work out what Luke wanted when he cried, but gradually I noticed that the cries were slightly different when he needed feeding, when he was cold or uncomfortable. I used to hate the sound of babies crying, but now I don't mind hearing Luke because I know he's trying to tell me something.'

Jan, 34, mother to Luke, 8 months

Responding to your baby's crying

▶ *Put your baby to your breast if you are breastfeeding – he may be hungry or want a cuddle.*

▶ *If you are bottle-feeding, is it time for a feed? If not, try giving him cooled boiled water.*

▶ *Check whether his nappy is wet or soiled.*

▶ *Wrap him up warmly and snugly – or if it is hot, try removing a layer of clothing.*

▶ *Try singing, music, rocking or a rhythmical noise, e.g. a loud, ticking clock in his room.*

▶ *Massage or gently rubbing his back, arms and legs can be soothing.*

▶ *Giving him a warm bath can be calming.*

▶ *Take him out for a walk in the pram/buggy during the day, or for a drive in the car at night.*

▶ *If you are busy doing housework, carry him around with you in a baby carrier or sling, preferably one which you wear on your front.*

▶ *If the crying seems incessant, leave him and make yourself a cup of tea.*

▶ *Before returning to him, take some deep breaths and 'think positive'.*

▶ *Phone a friend for support – or contact one of the dedicated support groups (see Taking it further).*

▶ *Ask a neighbour or friend to look after your baby for a while to give you a rest.*

▶ *Talk to your health visitor, doctor or post-natal supporter.*

▶ *Do not get upset if someone else is able to quieten him more easily than you.*

▶ *Take 'time out' for some relaxation and adult company.*

'Time out' for you and your partner

Once you have overcome the first couple of weeks, are getting to
know your baby and are beginning to find some semblance of order
from the initial chaos, it is time to think about your own needs and
having 'time out' – not just those precious ten minutes each day
but 'time *outside*', away from your baby. This is not only desirable;
it is essential. It helps you to maintain your sanity, reminds you
that you are an adult, ensures that you and your partner have time
together and will also prepare all of you for any future episodes
when you have to be apart for a while, for example, when you
return to work or if one of you is unwell. Remember, you started
as a couple and deserve to have time together as a couple, even
though time as a family is also beneficial.

Try to have the first occasion apart from your baby within the first
four to six weeks, then if possible, arrange to have one evening
out each week. It can be difficult the first time you leave your baby
with someone else, because you will be worried whether he will
be all right, whether he will miss you and whether your friend will
recognize his needs, but it is certain that your baby will be fine.
It may, of course, be of no benefit to any of you at this early stage
if your partner plans a romantic weekend away, as you are likely
to be too worried to enjoy it properly – save this for later. Initially,
arrange to do something just for an hour or two and stay fairly

local. You are then within reach if you are needed (unlikely), will not feel too beholden to your friend for looking after your baby and can return to collect him easily and quickly.

If you do not have friends or relatives locally, you will need to arrange a babysitter, but if finances are a problem, think about joining a babysitting circle – or form one of your own. This involves getting together a group of parents with small children who agree to babysit in return for some form of 'currency' that you agree between you. The currency may be curtain rings or counters, with each one being worth half an hour, and each family being given a set to start the circle going. You then pay with your curtain ring 'currency' but will later need to earn more by sitting for someone else, who repays you in curtain rings in return for your time. Alternatively, your 'currency' may be in the form of various tasks, each worth a certain amount of time, for example, mowing the lawn (partners), doing the shopping or ironing, or baking a birthday cake for a children's party.

If you are reading this while you are still pregnant, make a list of all the things that you and your partner like to do together, for example, walking in the park, going to the cinema or for a meal. Divide this list into activities that take a short period of time (up to three hours), those that take a medium length of time (up to a day) and those that take longer (holidays or weekends away), and keep the list handy for ideas once you have had your baby. Also think about some new things that you could do. Actively planning a date and time will commit you to going out and give you something to look forward to. Some ideas for maintaining your social life are given below.

Recreation ideas for new parents

▶ *Take a walk in the park, with your baby in the buggy or a sling.*
▶ *Arrange a cosy 'night in' with simple snacks, music and candles.*
▶ *Book a table at a restaurant or go to a country pub.*

(Contd)

- ▶ *Arrange to meet up with friends who have babies.*
- ▶ *Go to the cinema or rent a DVD.*
- ▶ *Set the dinner table in the garden and spend time after the meal talking to each other.*
- ▶ *Order a takeaway so you do not have to cook one evening each week.*
- ▶ *Play board games, do a crossword together or read to each other.*
- ▶ *Meet your partner near his workplace for lunch.*
- ▶ *Reserve seats for the theatre or a concert.*
- ▶ *Book a season ticket to attend sports games.*
- ▶ *Try to clear one day a week, perhaps at the weekend, when you can go out as a family, for a picnic, or shopping for something special (not the weekly food shopping).*

Returning to work

At some point, if you have taken maternity leave, you will have to decide whether or not to return to work, and if so, when. It is not an easy decision, whatever you had planned during your pregnancy, because your feelings may have changed dramatically since then. Your decision will, of course, depend on your family's financial situation, but may also be influenced by your occupation and seniority, whether you are employed or self-employed, the number of children in your family, whether you have a partner who is working and the practicalities of organizing your working day and childcare. Your partner, parents, in-laws and friends will also play a part, as will your social and cultural background and the support you have, both for yourself and your baby.

In order to make your decision, it may be useful to make a list for yourself, identifying the advantages and disadvantages of returning to work, balancing the positive financial, social and psychological benefits of working against the potential impact it may have on you, your baby and your partner. You may consider returning to work part-time, if this is permitted, but think about this very carefully. It will depend on the type of work you do, but you may find that you end up working full-time hours on part-time pay, or that part-time working adversely affects your chances of promotion or your pension. Ask for advice from your human resources department before starting your maternity leave, to find out whether there are tax or other implications of working part-time.

If you do decide to return to your job you will need to be even more organized, even earlier than if you decide to stay at home for several months or years to care for your child. You should, for example, put considerable effort into searching out a suitable person to care for your baby. Explore exactly which option is best for you, whether you decide to use a childminder, nursery, au pair, nanny, family member, or whether your partner chooses to stay at home to care for your baby. If you decide to pay someone outside the family, start searching during your pregnancy – it is never too early. In many areas childcare is both expensive and scarce and waiting lists are long. It can also take quite some time to find the person who is 'right' for you and your baby, whom you feel you can trust, who has similar views on caring for children to your own and who appears to relate well to babies (see Taking it further).

If you are breastfeeding, it can seem daunting to think of returning to work but it is not impossible. However, the earlier you return to work after the birth of your baby, the more difficult it can be, so it is wise to ensure that breastfeeding is well established before you need to work out how to manage everything. If you have the time, you can start expressing and freezing milk about a month before your return, so that you will have breast milk to leave with the person who is to care for your baby. You will also need to accustom your baby to feeding from a bottle, even if you are using expressed breast milk, and if you have decided to change from breast to artificial feeding, introduce this slowly. This gives your baby time to get used to the different milk and for his digestive system to adapt, and also allows your milk supply to reduce slowly, rather than stopping suddenly, when you will be more prone to engorged breasts. Similarly if you are going to use a mixed feeding system, in which your baby has artificial milk during your working hours and breast milk when you are home, this takes time for both of you to accept. You will need to think about whether you will express milk during your time at work to take home with you, how this can be done in privacy and where you will keep the milk until you leave for home.

> **Insight**
>
> Expressing milk means that you squeeze milk out of your breasts into a sterilized bottle, either by hand or, more commonly, by using a breast pump (manual or electric) which applies suction to your breast and mimics the action of the baby's mouth. The bottle can then be sealed and the milk frozen for up to a month.

Returning to work, and especially continuing to breastfeed at the same time, can be very tiring, even more so than staying at home to care for your baby. If you are someone who needs a lot of sleep and rest, it may not be best for you to return to work at this time – not only will you not be able to fulfil the requirements of your job but your own physical and emotional health may suffer from becoming excessively tired. When you first return to work, avoid arranging any major social events and if possible plan to return after having a holiday. If your company facilitates flexible working hours, use this option. Try to work out in advance whether you are essentially a 'morning person' or an 'evening person' – in other words, at what time of day are you at your most alert and awake? If you work better in the morning, perhaps you can arrange to work early in the day; if you work better in the afternoon or evening, try to organize starting and finishing later. Make sure you rest during your lunch break and go to bed early on the nights before your working days. On weekends or days off sleep as late as your home situation allows.

It is easy to feel guilty once you are a working mother. You may feel guilty and upset about leaving your child for someone else to look after, missing his first smile (or later, the seasonal concert at the nursery group), working when your parents think you should be at home with him, being late home to relieve the nanny, au pair or babysitter – and about a myriad of other small issues. However, *guilt is a wasted emotion*. It is natural to berate yourself but it will make no difference in most cases, so do not waste energy worrying about it, which will only serve to make you feel worse. If you continue to feel guilty about working, maybe it is not the best decision for you right now.

There are a few things you can do to help ease some of the reasons for feeling guilty. In the first few weeks, you may want to telephone the nursery or childminder all the time to check how your baby is coping, but after a while your 'working mind' will take over and you will not think of him so often, perhaps only when you are in the lavatory or when you stop for a coffee break. Recognize that the separation is usually worse for you than it is for your baby, especially in the first year, when he only needs to be fed, changed and to sleep. Make sure you are home every evening by a certain time so that you can bathe your baby or, later, read him a bedtime story. Arrange some 'back up' support for times when you are delayed, or your child carer is unavailable, and especially for occasions when your child is unwell. Keep a note in your diary of any special events involving your child, such as visits for immunizations, his first day at nursery or the local mother and baby group outing, and try to arrange not to work on those days. Provide your child carer with a camera to record notable moments, or ask her to send you a text picture on your mobile telephone.

If you have made a clear, logical and reasoned decision to return to work, think of all the positive things that this will bring for you, your baby and your family. To help put things in perspective, you may like to read Alison Pearson's book *I don't know how she does it* (Anchor, 2003). This is a marvellously hilarious account of a working mother's ups and downs, beginning with Kate, the heroine, standing in the kitchen at midnight distressing shop-bought mince pies to make them look like homemade ones, so that her small daughter will not feel embarrassed that her working mother has not had time to make any for the nursery school's Christmas party (and it does not take too long to read it either!).

> ## Top tip
> If you have decided to return to work, think of all the positive aspects it will bring. Enjoy it, and value the quality time you have with your baby when you are home. And remember – guilt is a wasted emotion, especially if you can do nothing about the situation.

10 THINGS TO REMEMBER

1 *Try to get organized during pregnancy so that housework is minimal when your baby is born.*

2 *If your partner is happy to share chores around the house, this does not have to mean that you each do 50 per cent of every chore – it may be easier to divide up the tasks and each do some of them.*

3 *Try to find time every day for yourself.*

4 *Work out ways of restricting visitors and telephone calls in the first few weeks of your baby's life.*

5 *Eat well and regularly to maintain your energy and to ensure that you are healthy enough to care for your baby.*

6 *Sleepless nights are a normal part of being a new parent – so rest when you can during the daytime.*

7 *Crying is your baby's way of communicating with you – learn to identify what the different types of crying mean.*

8 *Make sure you find time for you and your partner to have some time alone every week – even if it is just an hour.*

9 *Think through your options about returning to work – and if you change your mind after your baby is born, it does not matter.*

10 *Try not to feel guilty about your decisions as a parent – only you can know whether or not the decisions you make are right for you and your family.*

13

....

Physical well-being

In this chapter you will learn:
- *what physically happens to your body after delivery*
- *some strategies to help you recover from the birth*
- *factors to help you to feed your baby appropriately*
- *ways to regain and maintain your fitness.*

As well as paying attention to your emotional and social well-being, your body will need some time to recover from the birth and to return to normal, although this is never quite the same as before you were pregnant. All the parts of your body that changed to accommodate your growing baby will need to reduce in size, return to their usual position and your breasts need to prepare for lactation.

Your reproductive organs perhaps undergo the greatest change, as your uterus shrinks back into your pelvis and sheds the lining and any cells that are left from the placenta. This involves all the extra tissues, blood vessels, muscles and ligaments, which grew and developed during pregnancy, dissolving through a process of self-digestion and shrinking, called autolysis and involution, with the fluid being passed out in your urine – you will notice that you pass large quantities of urine in the first four or five days after the birth. Unfortunately, because there is so much extra fluid in your system, your kidneys cannot cope with it all at once, so some of the fluid moves elsewhere in your body, often making swollen ankles and fingers worse than when you were pregnant. This is normal and any swelling should disappear within a few days.

Insight

Urinary infections are common after delivery especially if the area is contaminated with blood. You may experience a burning sensation when passing urine, and will probably feel the need to go to the toilet much more often, yet will be unable to pass more than a tiny amount. You can begin to feel quite unwell with nausea, headaches and a temperature, so it is important to call your doctor if you feel like this. A urine specimen can be sent for analysis and the correct antibiotics prescribed.

You will also have a vaginal blood loss for some time after delivery, like a very heavy period, as any remaining tissues, together with the lining of the uterus, are passed out. These discharges are called *lochia* and are initially red and quite heavy for two or three days, then changing to brown for a further few days and eventually becoming a whitish or yellowish coloured discharge which can last a few days or up to a month after delivery. Sometimes you may pass large blood clots: inform your midwife or doctor, who may ask to see any sanitary pads you have saved to check whether the blood clots contain pieces of placenta.

Insight

The vaginal blood loss which occurs after your baby's birth should become progressively less in amount and lighter in colour. If the discharge stops suddenly or returns to frank red blood this may mean that there are still small pieces of placenta left inside, which can cause haemorrhage or infection if left untreated. You should report this to your midwife or doctor. Occasionally this may mean you having a D&C – a uterine scrape under anaesthetic – to remove the tissue.

Insight

It is really important to attend to personal hygiene after your baby's birth in order to avoid infections. In addition to your normal daily shower or bath you may need to wash 'down below' after using the toilet, especially after having your bowels open, as well as each time you change your

(Contd)

sanitary pad. Please note that tampons are not advised at this time as not only will they be uncomfortable, but there is an increased risk of toxic shock syndrome developing.

If you have had a vaginal tear or episiotomy in labour, you may have stitches or grazes in your perineum (the area between your vagina and anus), or your buttocks may be bruised, any of which can be uncomfortable at this time. Passing urine can increase this sensitivity as the slightly acid urine runs over your stitches or grazes. However, there are some things that you can do to ease the discomfort – see below.

Insight

If you have any stitches from a tear or episiotomy these will normally be dissolvable and do not need to be removed. However, occasionally a stitch may fail to dissolve and will need to be cut with scissors so that it can be removed. If you have any discomfort in the perineum or vagina after three or four weeks, inform your health visitor or doctor.

Caring for your perineum after delivery

Technique	How to use
Self-help techniques	• Keep the area scrupulously clean and dry to aid healing and prevent infection and change sanitary pads frequently.
	• Shower at least twice a day and wash down every time you have used the lavatory.
	• Eat a nourishing diet to aid wound healing, including foods containing zinc, iron, vitamins B and C; eat plenty of fresh fruit and vegetables and drink plenty of water (see also Chapter 5, Physical well-being).

Technique	How to use
Aromatherapy/ herbal remedies	• Essential oils of lavender and/or tea tree can be added to the bath water to prevent infection, ease discomfort and aid healing • Add to a jug of cooled boiled water and use it to wash down your perineum and vaginal opening after using the lavatory • Marigold and lavender, as well as comfrey, are wound healing plant remedies – consult a herbalist on how to use them • Witch hazel in a compress can be effective. • Calendula tablets can also aid healing.
Homeopathic/Bach flower remedies	• Rescue Remedy cream can be applied to sore buttocks but not directly to the wound area. • Crab apple Bach flower remedy is useful if you feel 'unclean'. • Homeopathic arnica tablets are renowned as a remedy for shock and bruising; arnica cream should not be applied directly to a wound. • Homeopathic hypericum can aid healing.

Your blood pressure, temperature, heart rate and breathing all return to normal within a day of two of delivery. Deep breathing encourages your lungs to inflate fully after having been compressed by the baby and your diaphragm in late pregnancy. Your blood clotting mechanism changes towards the end of pregnancy in an attempt to prevent excessive haemorrhage during labour, which means that you are more at risk of blood clots (thrombosis) in the early days after delivery. Getting up and about soon after your baby's birth and ensuring that you do ankle-circling exercises will help to prevent this but if you experience any discomfort in your calf, inform your midwife or doctor as soon as possible. Your digestive system can take a while to recover from pregnancy, and constipation in the early days is not uncommon; this is often compounded by the fear of discomfort when you have your bowels open for the first time after delivery. Some suggestions for dealing with post-natal constipation are given below.

> **Insight**
>
> Signs of a blood clot (thrombosis) in your leg include pain and redness, swelling and heat in one calf; sometimes the red area also feels lumpy to touch. If you experience these symptoms go to bed and call your doctor or midwife so that rapid treatment can be arranged (usually blood-thinning drugs).

Dealing with post-natal constipation

(See also Chapter 5, Constipation.)

Technique	How to use
Self-help techniques	• Privacy is a priority – give yourself time and space to sit on the lavatory in comfort without worrying that someone else may need the bathroom; lock the door if necessary.
	• Make sure your baby is asleep and unlikely to need you, take the phone off the hook and tell your partner and other children not to disturb you.
	• Take some deep breaths and try your relaxation exercises before starting to defecate.
	• If you have had haemorrhoids (piles) or your stitches are very painful, use some local anaesthetic gel around your anus just before attempting to have your bowels opened (ask your doctor/ midwife).

Technique	How to use
	• Do not strain or force yourself to pass a stool, try again later.
	• Ensure you drink at least two litres of water every day and eat plenty of fresh fruit, vegetables and other high fibre foods.
Massage and aromatherapy	• Firm, clockwise massage of your abdomen can stimulate the movement of your gut and encourage the passage of faeces towards your rectum.
	• Essential oils of mandarin, tangerine, sweet orange, bergamot, grapefruit or neroli, a total of four drops blended in 5 ml of grapeseed oil, can be used for abdominal massage or in the bath.
	• If your haemorrhoids are a problem, try sitting in cypress essential oil in the bath to constrict them; witch hazel is also good.

Feeding your baby

There are huge hormone changes in the early post-natal period, starting when your placenta is expelled just after your baby's birth. This causes a sudden drop in pregnancy hormones, especially oestrogen, which causes a corresponding release of the lactation hormone, prolactin, from the pituitary gland in your brain. Prolactin starts the process of milk production in the breast (see Figure 13.1); milk being made from the fatty globules in your blood. It is the action of putting your baby to your breast to suckle that triggers your 'let down' reflex in which oxytocin is released from your pituitary gland to stimulate special cells in the breast. These cells squeeze the milk-producing cells, causing milk to be forced towards the nipple. Suckling in turn stimulates more prolactin to produce more milk. Thus breastfeeding is very much a 'supply and demand' situation – the more your baby suckles, the more milk will be produced. Conversely, if you decide not to breastfeed your baby, or when you start to wean him onto solid foods, reducing the time he spends suckling at the breast decreases the prolactin supply and the consequent oxytocin stimulation, so milk production is also decreased.

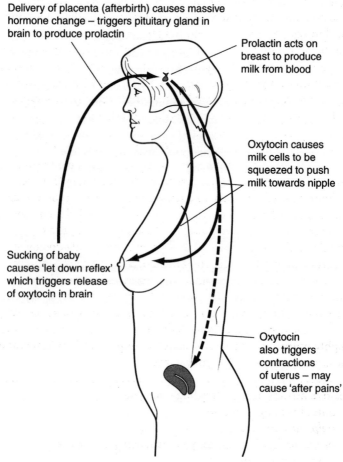

Delivery of placenta (afterbirth) causes massive hormone change – triggers pituitary gland in brain to produce prolactin

Prolactin acts on breast to produce milk from blood

Oxytocin causes milk cells to be squeezed to push milk towards nipple

Sucking of baby causes 'let down reflex' which triggers release of oxytocin in brain

Oxytocin also triggers contractions of uterus – may cause 'after pains'

Figure 13.1 Lactation process.

Milk production is a continuous cycle of supply and demand – the more you put your baby to the breast, the more milk you will produce.

During your pregnancy you will need to think about how you hope to feed your baby, but be prepared to keep an open mind. Everyone knows that breastfeeding is best for babies, since humans produce milk for human babies. Artificial (formula) milk is produced from cow's milk – but cow's milk is intended for calves, so it has to be changed in several ways to make it suitable for human consumption. However, breastfeeding does not suit all mothers and you may decide that you would prefer to bottle-feed your baby. If you and your partner have decided that breastfeeding does not appeal to you, or if you are returning to work soon after the birth, it can be more convenient and easier to establish than breastfeeding. If you have any medical conditions which could be made worse by the exertion of breastfeeding, such as a heart problem, or if you require medication which could be passed to your baby, you may be advised by your doctor or midwife to bottle-feed.

The following points aim to give you the positive aspects of breastfeeding *or* bottle-feeding but you will see that there are infinitely more advantages to the former, especially for your baby. It is not the aim of this section to try to influence your decision as it is your choice and may be based on very particular, personal circumstances. Whatever your reasons, you need to be happy – and positive – about the decision you make. Ask your midwife, family doctor or paediatrician for advice and sources of local information – and see Taking it further for some other suggestions. However, if you find it difficult to make a decision at this stage, it is worth trying breastfeeding first, even if it is only for a week or two, as the early milk, or colostrum, which your baby receives in the first few days, is highly nutritious and provides several important antibodies and protective mechanisms for your baby.

Positive aspects of breastfeeding – for you
- ▶ *aids shrinking of uterus*
- ▶ *helps weight loss*
- ▶ *hormone levels when fully breastfeeding may have contraceptive effect*
- ▶ *quick, easy, no preparation*
- ▶ *inexpensive*

(Contd)

- ▶ *less post-natal depression*
- ▶ *less risk of breast cancer*
- ▶ *less risk of ovarian cancer*
- ▶ *less risk of osteoporosis.*

Positive aspects of breastfeeding – for your baby
- ▶ *aids development of his immune system*
- ▶ *aids responses to vaccinations*
- ▶ *nutritional effects may enhance child's learning abilities at school*
- ▶ *aids social development*
- ▶ *better dental health*
- ▶ *better general health*
- ▶ *fewer digestive infections*
- ▶ *less diarrhoea*
- ▶ *fewer breathing problems*
- ▶ *less risk of eczema/allergy*
- ▶ *less risk of obesity*
- ▶ *less risk of diabetes*
- ▶ *less risk of high blood pressure*
- ▶ *less risk of cot death*
- ▶ *less risk of rheumatoid arthritis.*

Positive aspects of breastfeeding – for society
- ▶ *reduces cost of infant feeding*
- ▶ *reduces medical care costs*
- ▶ *helps child spacing*
- ▶ *increases survival of siblings*
- ▶ *more effective vaccination*
- ▶ *more ecological.*

Positive aspects of bottle-feeding – for you
- ▶ *offers you a choice*
- ▶ *easier to establish than breastfeeding, more convenient, more comfortable to establish*

Breastfeeding is the best and most natural way of providing your baby with all the nourishment he needs, but it can take some time to get lactation established. Unlike pregnancy, breastfeeding is the time when you *should* be eating for two! Eat plenty of protein foods, vitamins and minerals, fruit and vegetables, to prevent illnesses and infections (see Part 1, How to achieve a balanced diet), and drink *at least* two to three litres of fluid daily. Eating foods containing garlic, as well as nettle or fennel seed teas appears to aid milk supply; oats, perhaps eaten as porridge, may increase the duration of your baby's suckling. Breastfeeding can be tiring so try the Bach flower remedy, olive, two drops in water two or three times a day or as needed, and if you get frustrated try Rescue Remedy, four drops neat on your tongue (see also Part 4).

Make sure you are comfortable and in a suitable position before starting to breastfeed. Go to the lavatory to empty your bladder, and make sure any stitches do not feel too painful – take a mild painkilling tablet if necessary. Find a comfortable chair or sit propped up with pillows if you are on the bed. Bring your baby up to your breast rather than leaning down to him; use a pillow underneath him to support his weight; this avoids backache and pain in your neck or between your shoulder blades. Hold him closely with his face towards you in a straight line with his back so that his spine and neck do not arch.

His nose or top lip should be opposite your nipple and he should be able to reach your breast and nipple easily without having to twist or stretch. Always move your baby towards your breast rather than leaning your breast towards him. At night in bed, or if you have stitches or a Caesarean section wound which remains uncomfortable, try lying on your side with your baby lying facing you. Another way is to hold your baby with his body tucked under your arm, his feet pointing backwards and his head lying in your hand.

Wait until your baby opens his mouth wide enough to attach to your nipple; you may find it helpful to brush your nipple against his lips to encourage him to do this. Ask for help from your midwife or health visitor to ensure that your baby is fixed onto your breast correctly in order to prevent soreness and impaired milk supply. The easiest way to work this out for yourself is to suck your thumb! Note that your thumb points upwards and backwards towards the upper palate of your mouth. In order to suck your thumb properly it must be well inside your mouth; your tongue will be underneath your thumb so that you can suck. Now imagine that your thumb is your nipple within your baby's mouth – the nipple is directed upwards and backwards, his tongue will be underneath and all of your nipple and most of the darkened areola around the nipple should be inside his mouth, with his bottom lip as far away as possible from the base of your nipple. If your nipple is not in his mouth adequately, all he will do is to suck the end of it; you will become sore and he will get frustrated because he is not getting enough milk out. When he is properly attached to your breast, his mouth will be wide open and he will have a big mouthful of breast with his chin touching your breast and his bottom lip curled back. If you can see any of the areola (the brown skin around the nipple), there will be more visible above his top lip than below his bottom one. When he is feeding properly and taking in milk, you will note that his sucking pattern changes from short sucks to long deep sucks with little pauses in between. You may find *Succeed at Breastfeeding* (Hodder Education, 2010) a useful guide to breastfeeding your baby successfully.

In the early days, it is not uncommon for your nipples to become sore; if this happens, steep two camomile tea bags in boiling water, drain, cool and squeeze till no longer dripping but still moist, then place them in your bra over your nipples. Some commercial nipple creams also contain camomile, but wipe off excess cream before putting your baby to your breast. Geranium (pelargonium) leaves placed inside your bra with the underside of the leaves nearest to your skin, will also help to relieve soreness and reduce inflammation. If your breasts become engorged, swollen and painful, which is common when the milk first comes into the breast, at about four to five days, use dark green cabbage leaves, wiped clean and cooled in the refrigerator. (Do not wash them as this interferes with osmosis, which draws out the excess fluid.) Place the leaves inside your bra to reduce swelling, replace them when wet and keep repeating until you feel more comfortable. A simple reflexology technique to increase milk supply is to massage the areas between the knuckles of both hands; this area corresponds to the reflex zone for the breast (see Part 4). Gentle breast massage with both hands towards your nipples also encourages milk flow, but if you wish to use oils, avoid essential oils and use only a carrier oil to aid movement. Essential oils should not be applied to the breasts unless you scrupulously wipe them off before putting your baby to suckle, otherwise he will ingest them and they may affect his digestion.

Insight

Any stimulation of your breasts in the early weeks may cause a leakage of milk because of the 'supply and demand' effect. This includes rubbing or massaging your breasts, warmth from the atmosphere or from the shower or bath, sexual

(Contd)

stimulation – or simply hearing your baby's cry. This is normal but you may need to wear breast pads inside your bra when you are in public.

Homeopathic remedies can be helpful with breastfeeding problems, but it is important to choose one that most closely matches your symptoms. Use the 30C strength, one tablet 2–3 hourly as required. If you have had no response within five days, stop taking the remedy and consult a qualified practitioner. Phytolacca is suitable if you have excess milk, lumpy tender breasts and feel irritable; pulsatilla is appropriate for insufficient milk, cracked, burning nipples, tense, swollen breasts and if you keep crying and need sympathy. Chamomilla is better if the engorgement makes you feel so irritable that you cannot bear it and you get headaches after feeding (see Part 4 for more information).

Post-natal mobility

It is important to be up and about fairly soon after the birth, to avoid the risk of complications such as blood clots (thrombosis), chest infections and urinary problems, but you may find it difficult in the first few days to become very active. Your body is working hard, recovering from the birth, adapting to no longer being pregnant and establishing lactation. You will still feel heavy, cumbersome and uncomfortable for some time and may develop new aches and pains as a result of the labour. For example, neck and backache is not uncommon, especially if you have had a long second stage of labour, or after an epidural anaesthetic. Your spine, skeleton and the large muscles in your body take about a year to recover from pregnancy so exercise is essential to tone everything up. Your pelvic floor and anus have been stretched too during the delivery of your baby and it is vital to exercise this area (pelvic floor exercises, or Kegel exercises), to avoid urinary or faecal incontinence (leaking) when you cough, laugh or strain and, later in life, prolapse of your uterus. Also, although you will obviously lose some weight immediately after the birth of your baby, you may be surprised about how much you still have to lose. Gentle exercises in the first six weeks are encouraged to help tone up all the overstretched muscles in your body; later you can return to your normal exercise programme, or use this as an opportunity to start a regular exercise routine. There are several activities you can do which will aid your return to fitness if you do not wish or cannot get to an exercise class, and some suggestions are given below.

Post-natal exercises

Type of exercise	How to do it
Deep breathing to help inflate your lungs fully and prevent chest infections	• Once or twice each day, take ten deep controlled breaths – draw air into your lungs for as long as you can, hold for few seconds, then slowly let the air out.
Leg exercises to stimulate circulation and prevent thrombosis	• Whenever possible, circle each ankle several times one way then in the opposite direction.
Pelvic floor exercises to tighten muscles, aid circulation for healing, prevent incontinence and other problems later in life	• This exercise can be done anywhere and should be done several times daily, for the rest of your life: tighten up perineal muscles without tightening your buttock muscles, hold to a count of four and release. (NB: this is the same movement as if you are trying to stop passing urine, but do not do the exercises while passing urine as this increases the risk of infection.)

(Contd)

Type of exercise	How to do it
Abdominal exercises to tighten the band of muscles running down the middle of your abdomen – weeks one to six	• Kneeling on all fours with your back flat, pull your tummy towards your spine to tighten your abdominal muscles, hold and release; repeat ten times. • Lying on your back, knees bent, feet flat on floor, breathe in, squeeze abdominal muscles and flatten the small of your back towards the floor, hold and release; repeat ten times (pelvic tilt).
Abdominal exercises from week six onwards (plus earlier exercises, above)	• Lying on your back, knees bent, feet on floor, hands resting on thighs, breathe in; as you breathe out, pull in abdominal muscles and slide hands up thighs towards knees, lifting head and shoulders off the floor; hold at the highest most comfortable point, but do not strain; release; repeat ten times. • Lying on back, knees bent, feet on floor, tighten abdominal muscles, keeping small of back in neutral position; slide legs away from body until knees are straight, using abdominal muscles to prevent small of back from arching; repeat ten times. • On all fours, knees hip-width apart and hands at least shoulder-width apart, keep back flat, abdominal muscles pulled in; bend elbows and push chin towards floor, straighten up; repeat ten times.

'I found my pelvic floor exercises difficult to do, especially in the first few days. Quite apart from remembering them and finding time to do them, I couldn't actually feel what I was supposed to be doing, as I'd had an episiotomy and was very bruised underneath.'

Kate, 19, mother to Sam, 4 months

Post-natal fitness

There are many types of exercise that will stimulate your cardiovascular system, your circulation and breathing and help you to maintain a healthy heart, as well as toning muscle groups for better posture and overall well-being. If you do not wish or are unable to join a formal fitness class or local gymnasium, there are many informal ways of increasing your fitness and health.

Informal ways of improving fitness
- *breastfeeding – aids weight loss*
- *walking in the park with your baby*
- *vacuuming*
- *dancing and singing to music while doing household chores*
- *gardening, mowing the lawn*
- *walking up escalators in shops (if you do not have the buggy!)*
- *walking to local shops every day instead of driving to the supermarket*
- *swimming after your baby's swimming class*
- *buy a mini trampoline – great for your pelvic floor and abdominals.*

Suggestions for your fitness programme
- *pilates, yoga*
- *swimming, water-based exercises*
- *cycling – whole family can join in*
- *aerobic exercise*
- *horse riding*
- *dancing – salsa, ballroom, line, etc.*

- *weight training (build up slowly)*
- *getting advice from personal fitness trainer.*

You will also, no doubt, be keen to lose the weight you have gained during pregnancy, but it is important to tackle this slowly. Regular exercise will help you to tone up and lose weight but you may not return to your 'normal' weight for some time, especially if you are breastfeeding (in some women all the weight is lost after they stop breastfeeding, but it is recognized that the longer you breastfeed the more weight you will lose). It can certainly take a good six months for you to lose the weight and you should aim to lose no more than half a kilogram per week. Calorie counting is definitely not recommended if you are breastfeeding as you need about an extra 500 calories a day during this time, and even if you are bottle-feeding, your body still needs time to adjust slowly. Eat nourishing healthy meals, take regular gentle exercise and be patient. If you encourage your partner and children to eat healthily and to exercise as well it will be much easier; taking your baby/toddler to activities which promote a variety of exercises for children will also help everyone to develop habits for healthy living.

10 THINGS TO REMEMBER

1 *Breastfeeding is the most natural way to feed your baby and it's also best for you.*

2 *Ask your midwife for help with breastfeeding. They can help to fix your baby on the breast properly to avoid sore nipples.*

3 *Breastfeeding works on a 'supply and demand' principle – the more you put your baby to your breast the more milk you will produce.*

4 *If you have excessive vaginal bleeding after the birth or very large blood clots, or if bleeding continues for more than three weeks, inform your midwife or doctor.*

5 *You will pass copious amounts of urine immediately after the birth, but report any burning sensations which could mean a urine infection.*

6 *Eat well to ensure that you return to good health in order to have the energy to care for your baby, and to provide nourishment for your baby when breastfeeding.*

7 *Do NOT expect to be back to your pre-pregnancy shape and size immediately after your baby's birth.*

8 *Performing regular daily pelvic floor exercises is the best way of regaining your muscle tone, which is good for your sex life, and for preventing incontinence of urine or faeces.*

9 *Rest when you can in order to conserve your energy, but start gentle exercise fairly soon, e.g. walking to the park.*

10 *If you wish to return to, or start, more formal physical exercise do inform your instructor that you have recently had a baby.*

Part four

Positive complementary therapies

14

Using complementary therapies safely in pregnancy and childbirth

In this chapter you will learn:
- *how to take homeopathic remedies appropriately in pregnancy*
- *how to use aromatherapy safely in pregnancy and childbirth*
- *the safe use of herbal medicines*
- *how to self-administer Bach flower remedies*
- *definitions of other commonly used complementary therapies.*

Complementary therapies are increasingly being used during pregnancy and childbirth, both by expectant mothers who purchase natural remedies such as aromatherapy oils, herbal, homeopathic and Bach flower remedies from health stores, and by professionals, especially midwives and doulas, to enhance the care they provide. However, it is vital to appreciate that, just because these therapies are 'natural' they are not automatically also 'safe' – they *must* be used appropriately and accurately. This section provides a summary of how to use some of the most commonly used remedies and a glossary of terms of some of the other therapies mentioned in this book. If you have any doubts about either the safety or effectiveness of any complementary therapy treatments you may be having, or about natural remedies you are taking, it is wise to seek professional advice first – see Taking it further.

How to take homeopathic remedies in pregnancy

Homoeopathy is an energy-based system of complementary medicine in which minute doses of various substances are used to treat conditions whereas, if the same substances were given in large quantities, they would actually cause the same symptoms (often referred to as 'treating like with like'). The remedy must be matched precisely to the full set of symptoms of each individual. There is little direct research on homeopathy in pregnancy but many women have used it successfully to ease pregnancy symptoms and to help them through labour and early parenthood, although it is wise to consult a qualified practitioner for the most appropriate treatment.

Homeopathic remedies do not work in the same way as drugs and will not interfere with them, although some medicines, such as certain strong antibiotics, can prevent the homeopathic remedies from working effectively. It is important to select the most appropriate remedy as incorrect use can trigger new symptoms, while failing to treat your original symptoms. Choose a remedy which best suits your particular symptoms (from the suggested remedies in each section of this book) and try it for five days. If you have had no response at all after five days, it is probably the wrong remedy and you should not take it any longer, as occasionally it may actually cause new symptoms to develop, making you feel even worse. You may experience a 'healing crisis' when you first start taking the remedy, in which you get a temporary worsening of your symptoms; this often indicates that you have chosen the correct remedy and the feeling should pass within 24 hours, after which time you should start to feel better.

Avoid eating, drinking or smoking for about 15 minutes before and after taking each remedy and change your toothpaste to a fruit-flavoured one while you are taking the remedies as some do not work when you use mint-flavoured paste. You should also limit the amount of coffee you drink (a good idea in pregnancy anyway), as this can stop some of the remedies from working effectively. If you are taking any medications, especially some painkillers, antibiotics, antacids, tablets for a fungal infection or blood thinning drugs (anticoagulants), you may find that the homeopathic remedy does not relieve your symptoms.

In most shops you will find the remedies available in two strengths – 6C and 30C – the 30C strength is likely to be more effective. You should try taking one tablet, under your tongue, every two or three hours. Stronger doses, such as 200C, are usually only available from specialist homeopathic pharmacies – see Taking it further. Tip them directly into the lid of the bottle and then into your mouth, or onto your clean hand. Do not put them onto a metal spoon or let other people handle them, as the tablets may not work. You may need to change your remedy as your symptoms change.

Arnica is a commonly used homoeopathic remedy to treat bruising, shock and trauma, especially painful stitches, after your baby's birth. Take one 30C strength tablet as soon as possible after the birth, then one tablet three times daily for three days, then stop. Arnica cream is useful if your buttocks are bruised but should not be applied directly over the stitches.

Safe use of aromatherapy in pregnancy and childbirth

Aromatherapy is the use of highly concentrated plant oils, usually administered in massage or in the bath. Aromatherapy and massage can be extremely relaxing and may ease symptoms in pregnancy such as backache, constipation, headache, anxiety and stress.

However, all aromatherapy essential oils contain chemicals which give them their specific therapeutic properties (e.g. relaxing, uplifting or stimulating) and once absorbed into the body they work in exactly the same way as drugs – so *do not* assume that they are all safe in pregnancy and labour. Many oils should not be used at all in pregnancy as the molecules cross the placenta to the baby. As a general rule, avoid using any oils in the first three months, unless you have been advised by an expert, as it is not known exactly how the oils can affect you or your baby. If you have any medical or pregnancy-related problems, do not use aromatherapy until you have checked with your midwife or doctor that it is safe to do so. After the birth, it is unwise to use essential oils at all on your baby until he is at least three months old as they may irritate the skin or, more importantly, interfere with the continuing development of his immune system.

The oils considered the safest in pregnancy are the citrus oils, which are uplifting and refreshing (for example, orange, grapefruit, lime, bergamot and neroli/orange blossom), as well as ylang ylang, which is a very relaxing oil that can lower blood pressure, and frankincense, an extremely calming and balancing oil. Most other oils should be used with care – even lavender needs to be used cautiously as there are various types, each containing different chemicals, some of which are safe and others which may not be.

Do not be tempted to buy essential oils from local markets or high street shops that do not specialize in good quality health products. The oils should be pure, although it is not necessary to buy organic oils unless you particularly want to. When you buy them, they should not be ready-blended with other oils including base/carrier oils such as grapeseed or sweet almond – always buy this separately. The range of oils should be of varying prices – beware any high street shop in which all the oils are more or less the same price. Some oils are very expensive because of the specialist methods needed to extract the oils from the plants – rose, neroli and jasmine are the most expensive, but frankincense, ylang ylang and sandalwood are also quite costly. Concentrated essential oils should always be in small dark glass bottles as they deteriorate in the presence of oxygen, light and other chemicals such as plastic. Most have a 'sell by' date, although this is not always on the bottle, but generally, citrus oils last only six months and should be kept in the refrigerator, while most others will last up to two years. Do not store your essential oils in the same place as your homeopathic remedies, which can be inactivated by strong smelling substances.

Always blend your essential oils in a carrier oil, even if you are putting them in the bath, to avoid them coming into contact with the skin neat. Grapeseed is probably the best carrier, but peach kernel, sweet almond (unless you are allergic to almonds), safflower oil and several others can also be used. Do not use baby oil, which is usually a mineral oil and will not absorb into the skin. For massage you can use a maximum of two drops to each 5 ml (teaspoon) of carrier oil – so if you want to use several essential oils together you will need to use more carrier oil. Try not to use more than three essential oils in one blend. In the bath you can add five to six drops to a teaspoon of carrier (or full cream milk if you prefer) and drop this into the bath while the hot water is running. Remember that, irrespective of the way in which you administer the oils, you will be inhaling the vapours as well and the chemicals from the inhaled vapours pass to your lungs and then via your bloodstream to the rest of your body. If you like to use a vaporizer or steam dispenser at home, do not leave it on for more than 10–15 minutes in each hour – and never leave it on all night in a bedroom.

Aromatherapy can be particularly useful during labour as the essential oils used are thought to contain chemicals which are pain-relieving, relaxing and which may encourage the uterus to work more efficiently. The aromas can be pleasantly distracting – but be aware that they can also seem heavy and cloying if used continuously, giving you (and your partner and midwife!) a headache or making you feel sick. Certain oils need to be used with care and only after discussion with your midwife who can explain how far your labour has progressed and whether it is appropriate to use them – this applies specifically to oils that may increase contractions such as clary sage and jasmine. Some midwives use aromatherapy, but if you wish to use your own oils, do tell your midwife what you are doing so that she can plan the rest of your care accordingly, to avoid complications, as some of the oil chemicals can interfere with prescribed drugs you may need. If you wish to be accompanied in labour by a private aromatherapist, discuss this with your midwives in advance, particularly if you are having your baby in hospital or a birth centre.

Guidelines for using aromatherapy oils in labour

- ▶ *Use two drops of essential oil in 5 ml of carrier oil, e.g. grapeseed, for massage.*
- ▶ *Use four drops of essential oil in 5 ml carrier oil for baths.*
- ▶ *Add two drops of essential oil in a vaporizer and use for only 10–15 minutes in each hour.*

- ▶ Do not add oils to the birthing pool if your waters have broken.
- ▶ Ask someone to massage your feet, shoulders and abdomen with diluted oils.
- ▶ Use oils in a foot bath if you prefer not to be touched.
- ▶ Make a compress with a towel soaked in water with four drops of essential oil, to put over the small of your back, pubic area or shoulders.
- ▶ Lavender and rose oils ease pain and relax you.
- ▶ Ylang ylang, lavender and marjoram oils lower blood pressure.
- ▶ Jasmine and clary sage oils enhance contractions, but use with care and only after discussion with your midwife.
- ▶ Grapefruit, bergamot, tangerine and sweet orange oils are uplifting.
- ▶ Spearmint or peppermint oils ease nausea.
- ▶ A single drop of frankincense oil, massaged very lightly and slowly into the centre of your palm, is calming especially as you approach second stage (transition).

Safe use of herbal remedies in pregnancy

Herbal medicine (medical herbalism) is the use of plants for their therapeutic properties. They act inside your body in exactly the same way as drugs and may therefore compete with any medications you may need. Many herbal remedies are contraindicated in pregnancy so it is important *always* to consult an expert and to avoid the routine use of any herbal medicines during pregnancy. Inform your midwife or doctor about *any* herbal remedies or teas you are taking in pregnancy and avoid all herbal medicines in the first three months when your baby's major organs are developing. Only take herbal remedies if you have a specific issue you wish to address, only if you know that they are safe to use and only for a few weeks at most. It is not, for example, necessary to drink raspberry leaf tea routinely in pregnancy (often taken to tone the uterus for labour) if you have previously had a normal labour and delivery without any problems, since herbal remedies can sometimes adversely affect your body's ability to work efficiently. Stop taking all herbal remedies at least two weeks before any planned surgery, including Caesarean section.

Ginger is not the most appropriate, nor the safest, remedy for all women with 'morning sickness' as it can interfere with your body's blood-clotting mechanism. If you have nausea and vomiting and wish to try it, do not take it continuously for more than five days if you have no response, or if it makes you feel worse. Even if it is effective, do not take it for more than three weeks without a break, or ask your doctor to do a blood test to check your blood-clotting factors.

If you develop any unusual symptoms either during or after taking herbal medicines, inform your doctor; keep remedies out of reach of young children, but in the event of accidental administration, ensure that you inform your doctor or emergency service personnel which herbal remedy has been taken. The Medical Toxicology Unit at Guy's Hospital in London collates data about the adverse effects of drugs and other substances including a growing body of evidence on the dangers of herbal remedies. Although this is a service for healthcare professionals, it can be useful to know about it in the event that someone experiences problematic side effects from taking herbal remedies – see Taking it further.

Bach flower remedies for pregnancy and childbirth

Bach flower remedies are liquid plant essences, thought to have a positive effect on your emotions. There are 38 remedies plus the Rescue Remedy, a universal first aid/stress reliever, available. They are similar in principle to homeopathic remedies, although they are prepared differently, but as with homeopathy, they do not have a chemical action on your body in the same way as drugs and medicines and are considered safe to take in pregnancy. Remedies are preserved in brandy, so do not take them if you have moral or health reasons for avoiding alcohol. If, after taking them for some time, you still feel emotionally unwell, consult your midwife or doctor for further help, as you may benefit from more in-depth counselling. It is usual to take a short course of about two weeks, using two drops of the remedy dissolved in spring water, either three or four times daily – but this will depend on your particular symptoms and your reasons for using the remedies. Rescue Remedy is usually given as four drops, either neat on your tongue or in water, as required to combat stress, anxiety and panic, and can be taken as often as you need.

Bach flower remedy	Useful if you...	Bach flower remedy	Useful if you...
Agrimony	feel miserable but put on a 'brave' face	Crab apple	feel unclean, have a poor body image, especially after delivery
Aspen	feel frightened but don't know why	Elm	feel overwhelmed by work and responsibility
Beech	are critical, a perfectionist	Gentian	are depressed, pessimistic, as after a setback
Centaury	are not able to say 'no' – taking	Gorse	feel despairing and discouraged
Cerrato	constantly seek reassurance	Heather	are completely self-absorbed, have to keep talking about how you feel

(Contd)

Bach flower remedy	Useful if you...	Bach flower remedy	Useful if you...
Cherry plum	feel angry, fear you'll lose control	Holly	feel 'hard done by' or victimized
Chestnut bud	fail to learn from previous experiences	Honeysuckle	have feelings of nostalgia, live in past memories
Chicory	are overprotective	Hornbeam	experience that 'Monday morning feeling'
Clematis	are absent-minded, easily bored	Impatiens	are impatient and irritable, e.g. with premenstrual tension
Larch	lack self-confidence, doubt your own abilities	Star of Bethlehem	are shocked after a major trauma or bereavement
Mimulus	fear something specific, e.g. labour	Sweet chestnut	feel complete despair, unbearable unhappiness
Mustard	are depressed, gloomy for no known reason	Vervain	have pushed yourself too far

Bach flower remedy	Useful if you...	Bach flower remedy	Useful if you...
Oak	feel exhausted, overwhelmed by responsibility	Vine	are determined, tend to try to control people
Olive	are physically and mentally exhausted, weary – good in labour	Walnut	need help to adapt to the changes in your life, especially with a new baby
Pine	feel guilty	Water violet	are shy, private person, isolated
Red chestnut	worry excessively	White chestnut	experience unwanted thoughts going round your head
Rock rose	feel terrified, panic or suffer nightmares	Wild oat	need help to make changes in direction
Rock water	are a perfectionist, strong-willed	Wild rose	tend to drift, need some 'grounding'
Scleranthus	are unable to make decisions, perhaps whether or not to have amniocentesis	Willow	are full of self-pity, resentment or bitterness

10 THINGS TO REMEMBER

1 *Just because complementary therapies are 'natural',
   this does not mean that they are always safe, especially
   in pregnancy.*

2 *If in doubt about the safety of a particular complementary
   therapy or natural remedy, contact your midwife or
   www.expectancy.co.uk.*

3 *Some natural remedies, e.g. herbal medicines and
   aromatherapy oils, act in the same way as medical drugs
   and may interfere with any medications prescribed by
   your doctor.*

4 *Some natural remedies, e.g. homeopathic and Bach flower
   remedies, are types of energy medicine and may be inactivated
   by medical drugs or other substances.*

5 *Touch therapies, e.g. massage, aromatherapy, reflexology
   or shiatsu, can aid relaxation, reduce stress hormones and
   increase positive pregnancy and labour hormones.*

6 *When consulting a complementary therapist, ask them
   for evidence of their training and insurance cover to treat
   pregnant women.*

7 *ALWAYS inform your midwife and/or doctor that you are
   using complementary therapies or natural remedies.*

8 *It is particularly essential to inform your midwife if you wish
   to seek complementary therapies to start labour if you are past
   your due date.*

9   *If you wish to use complementary therapies in labour or be accompanied in labour by an independent practitioner or a doula who uses complementary therapies, you should discuss this with your midwife in advance.*

10 *If in doubt about the safety or effectiveness of a particular complementary therapy, do not use it until you have obtained expert advice.*

Glossary of complementary therapies

This glossary provides an overview of some of the other most commonly used complementary therapies and natural remedies in the UK and USA.

acupressure An aspect of Chinese medicine in which pressure is applied to various points on the body to stimulate or sedate internal energies; it has been used successfully to treat sickness in pregnancy, to speed up contractions and to relieve pain in labour.

acupuncture An aspect of Chinese medicine based on the principle of energy lines (meridians) linking different parts of the body to each other. Ill health or physical, emotional or spiritual stress may cause blockages or excesses of energy at certain points – needles are inserted into specific points along the meridians to rebalance energy flow and assist in a return to full health. It has been used to treat various pregnancy problems such as backache and indigestion, to relieve labour pain and for Caesarean section.

Alexander technique A method of re-educating people to change habitual posture and body movement to improve mobility, balance and coordination; can be used during pregnancy to ease physical symptoms such as backache and shoulder pain.

chiropractic A manual therapy based on the idea that the skeleton is the body's main supporting framework, with all soft parts of the body attached either inside or outside this framework; trauma, injury or disease cause strain and tension, triggering discomforts and disease. Treatment involves manipulation to re-align the spine and its relationship with the rest of the body. Chiropractic is effective in treating various pregnancy problems, e.g. backache, carpal tunnel syndrome, indigestion, sickness and for treating colic in babies, hyperactivity in children, as well as menstrual and menopausal symptoms in non-pregnant women.

....

counselling A consultation and discussion process in which the counsellor listens and helps you to solve problems through increased awareness and exploration of any difficulties you are experiencing or have previously experienced, so that you can make appropriate decisions and your life can be approached with more confidence and assertiveness.

....

craniosacral therapy A form of osteopathy using very gentle manipulation of the skull to release tension; successfully used to treat babies who are irritable after a difficult birth, and colic and hyperactivity in older children (see also **osteopathy**).

....

hypnotherapy Hypnosis is a therapeutic system used to cause changes in behaviour through a trance-like state of deep relaxation. Conditions which respond well include habits such as smoking, bed wetting in children or severe anxiety states; it has also been used successfully to help with labour pain and even to relax mothers sufficiently to turn their breech babies to head-first.

....

massage A systematic stroking or kneading of various parts of the body to aid relaxation, stimulate circulation and excretion (e.g. in constipation) and to lower blood pressure; it may be helpful for anxiety and fear in pregnancy and for relieving pain in labour, because touch impulses reach the brain quicker than pain impulses.

....

moxibustion A Chinese technique involving the burning of moxa sticks made from the herb mugwort, and used as a heat source when held over appropriate acupuncture points; an increasingly popular as a way of turning breech babies to head-first (see Chapter 9).

osteopathy A manual technique similar to chiropractic, in which manipulation of the skeleton, muscles, joints and ligaments helps to restore structure and function within the body; it may be effective in treating pregnancy sciatica, symphysis pubis pain and carpal tunnel syndrome (wrist tingling).

Qi gong A Chinese healing art using a series of gentle focused exercises for mind and body aimed at encouraging the body's vital life energy (Qi) to flow smoothly throughout the body.

reflexology, reflex zone therapy A manual therapy in which the feet (or hands) represent a map of the whole body: working on the feet means that other parts of the body can be treated; it appears to be especially good for relaxation, high blood pressure and problems such as constipation in pregnancy, stimulating contractions in labour and promoting a good milk supply after the birth of the baby.

shiatsu A manual therapy, similar to acupuncture, developed in Japan in the 1950s, involving thumb and finger pressure applied to specific points on your body; useful for 'morning sickness', promoting contractions in labour and easing colic in babies.

t'ai chi Similar to Qi gong – a series of slow, focused and relaxed exercises and movements performed in a special sequence with the aim of improving or maintaining health and well-being.

Conclusion

Have a Happy Pregnancy has offered you an opportunity to explore some of the numerous pregnancy and childbirth issues which you may have considered when you were planning to start or continue your family, and during those early weeks when you may not have felt at your best. It is hoped that you have been able to come to some decisions about the various aspects of your care, or that, by using the Taking it further section, you will begin to seek out those answers for yourself.

Pregnancy, birth and new motherhood is an exciting but confusing and worrying time and it is sometimes difficult to know where to turn for help. The maternity services can often seem overwhelming, particularly if you have no previous experience of medical care; and many hospitals are so busy that you may feel as if you are on a 'conveyor belt' being processed. There is not always adequate time or opportunity for you to think of all the questions you wish to ask, leaving you to go away still worrying or frightened about this momentous life event. It is easy to feel out of control when your life has been 'taken over' by your baby, both antenatally and after the birth, but the better prepared you are, the more confident you will feel. Knowledge is power and an awareness of what is happening gives you a greater sense of security and confidence to progress through the various stages of your pregnancy, labour and early days with your new baby.

Take each step one at a time and do not try to tackle too much in one go. Ask questions as much as you can – and make sure you feel comfortable with the answers. Tackle worries and problems as they arise and do not leave them untended, otherwise they will assume gigantic proportions in your mind. Try to be as assertive as possible so that you get the care you want. This is *your* childbirth experience and you deserve to get the one you want, or as near to it as your individual circumstances allow. Stay calm and focused and develop a positive attitude to the whole event, which will help you to enjoy your pregnancy, your baby's birth and the early days at home with him. Remember – think positive!

Taking it further

Of course, there are numerous books available on the subjects of pregnancy, birth and early parenthood, but there are also many websites that can be helpful. In today's technological age, it seems appropriate here to include Internet sites instead of books, as they will be regularly and more quickly updated and can usually point you in the direction of other sites and sources of information. There are literally hundreds of websites available but those listed below have been personally investigated and are recommended by the author of *Have a Happy Pregnancy*.

www.adviceguide.org.uk
Citizens Advice Bureau guide to benefits for families

www.aims.org.uk
Association to Improve Maternity Services

www.ainsworths.com
Ainsworth's Homeopathic Pharmacy – international mail-order service for homeopathic remedies

www.apec.org.uk
Action Against Pre-eclampsia (pregnancy high blood pressure syndrome)

www.apni.org
Association for Post-natal Illness (post-natal depression)

www.arc-uk.org
Antenatal Results and Choices – information and support on antenatal tests and investigations

www.ash.org.uk
Action on Smoking and Health

www.apdt.co.uk
Association of Pet Dog Trainers – offers courses on animal behaviour, including classes on preparing for or coping with a new addition to the family

www.avert.org/pregnancy
Averting HIV and AIDS

www.babycaretens.com
BabyCare TENS – hire and sale of transcutaneous electrical nerve stimulation apparatus for labour

www.babycentre.com
Comprehensive information for parents (also www.babycentre. co.uk)

www.babyfriendly.org.uk/page.asp?page=95
Baby Friendly Initiative downloadable leaflets for parents, on breast and bottle-feeding, available in 18 languages

www.babysittercircle.co.uk
Baby Sitter Circle – tips on setting up your own babysitting circle, how to obtain babysitting services online

www.bachcentre.com
Dr Edward Bach Flower Centre – information, advice and mail order

www.bacp.co.uk
British Association for Counselling and Psychotherapy – main UK organization related to counselling and psychotherapy, provides a register of practitioners

www.birthdefects
Birth Defects Research for Children

www.birthlight.com
Birthlight Trust promotes holistic approach to pregnancy and childbirth, specializing in yoga

www.birthtraumaassociation.org.uk
Birth Trauma Association for women with childbirth-related post traumatic stress disorder

www.bondpearcepersonalinjury.co.uk/Birth-Injury
Bond Pearce Personal Injury Solicitors – experienced at dealing with medical negligence claims for birth-related injuries to mother or baby

www.bpas.org.uk
British Pregnancy Advisory Service (unwanted pregnancy)

www.breastfeeding.com/helpme
Help for mothers who are breastfeeding

www.bso.ac.uk
British School of Osteopathy, London – has a specialist Expectant Mothers' Clinic run by senior student osteopaths with a supervising senior tutor and a midwife in attendance

www.chatas.co.uk
Child Health Alternative Therapy Advisory Service – offers independent advice to parents wanting to use complementary therapies for children, specializes in hypnosis for treatment of enuresis (bed wetting)

www.childbirth-massage.co.uk
Childbirth Essentials – offers the award-winning LK Massage Programme™ for couples preparing for labour, plus DVD for home use

www.childcarelink.gov.uk
Childcare Link – information and sources of help for childcare

www.childline.org.uk
Helpline for children who are victims of bullying

www.cre.gov.uk
Commission for Racial Equality

www.cry-sis.org
Support for parents with babies who cry continuously

www.deafparent.org.uk
Deaf Parenting UK

www.diabetes.co.uk/diabetes-and-pregnancy
Diabetes website – information on pregnancy and birth

www.disabledparentsnetwork.org.uk
Disabled Parents' Network

www.dsa-uk.com
Down's Syndrome Association

www.eoc-law.org.uk
Equal Opportunities Commission – detailed information on
maternity and parental rights

www.epilepsynse.org.uk/pages/info/leaflets/preg.cfm
National Society for Epilepsy – information on epilepsy related to
pregnancy and parenting

www.expectancy.co.uk
Expectant Parents' Complementary Therapies Consultancy –
information on safe use of complementary therapies in pregnancy
and childbirth, specialist 'morning sickness', breech and pregnancy
support consultations by telephone (UK, fee payable), and online
(international, free of charge), and on CD ROM; register of midwives
and Birth Support Therapists who use complementary therapies

www.fathersdirect.com
Fathers Direct – information and support for expectant fathers

www.fedant.org
Federation of Antenatal Educators – to help you find registered
teachers of antenatal classes, as well as insured doulas and
complementary practitioners

www.fpa.org.uk
Family Planning Association

www.foresight.gov.uk
Foresight – Association for Preconception Care

www.gcc-uk.org
General Chiropractic Council (UK) – registers of qualified chiropractors

www.gingerbread.org.uk
Gingerbread – support for lone parents

www.gbss.org.uk
Group B Strep. Support

www.helios.co.uk
Helios Homeopathic Pharmacy – provides advice and mail-order service of homeopathic remedies

www.herpes.com/pregnancy
Herpes information and support website

www.herpes-coldsores.com
Information on various sexually transmitted diseases

www.hse.gov.uk/mothers
Health and Safety Executive – information for expectant and new mothers

www.homebirth.org.uk
Home birth reference site

www.hyperemesis.org
Hyperemesis Education and Research (excessive 'morning sickness')

www.independentmidwives.org.uk
Independent Midwives Association (private home births)

www.lalecheleague.org.uk
La Leche League – help for breastfeeding mothers

www.medtox.org/chi
Medical Toxicology Unit at Guy's Hospital in London – special service for professionals with information on adverse effects from medicines including western and Chinese herbal medicines

www.meetamum.co.uk
Meet a Mum Association for those feeling isolated at home with a new baby

www.midwivesonline.com
Information for expectant mothers and fathers

www.miscarriageassociation.org.uk
Miscarriage Association

www.morningwell.co.uk
Morningwell™ – audio CD to help 'morning sickness', especially good if symptoms are made worse by movement, such as in the car

www.motherisk.org
Canadian website providing excellent information for parents about medical conditions in pregnancy and babies' and children's health

www.natalhypnotherapy.co.uk
Provides courses and CDs to help empower and relax pregnant women

www.ncma.org
National Childminding Association

www.nct.org
National Childbirth Trust – charitable organization

www.nspcc.org.uk
National Society for the Prevention of Cruelty to Children

www.nutritionaltherapycouncil.org.uk
Nutritional Therapy Council, the regulatory organization for
nutritional therapy

www.oneparentfamilies.org.uk
National Council for One Parent Families

www.osteopathy.org.uk
General Osteopathic Council – maintains register of qualified
osteopaths

www.pelvicpartnership.org.uk
Pelvic Partnership – support, information and advice for women
with pregnancy symphysis pubis discomfort/pelvic girdle pain

www.positivelywomen.org.uk
Information, support and advocacy for women with HIV

www.post-natalexercise.co.uk/mothers
Guild of Pregnancy and Post-natal Exercise Instructors –
information for mothers on exercise before and after childbirth

www.quit.org
NHS Pregnancy Smoking support

www.relate.org.uk
Relate – offers advice and counselling for individuals and couples
on both relationship and sexual problems

www.safemotherhood.org
Safe Motherhood Initiative (WHO international childbirth safety)

www.sheilakitzinger.com/BirthCrisis
Birth Crisis Network – UK telephone helpline for women wanting
to discuss a traumatic birth

www.sids.org.uk
Foundation for the Study of Infant Deaths

www.surestart.gov.uk
Sure Start – UK government programme aimed at facilitating the best start in life for every child, through information, childcare and family support

www.uk-sands.org
Stillbirth and Neonatal Death Society

www.ursulajames.co.uk
Respected hypnotherapist and lecturer with special interest in women's health issues

www.tamba.org.uk
Twins and Multiple Births Association

www.tommys.org
Tommy's the Baby Charity – information on miscarriage, premature birth and stillbirth

www.waterbirth.co.uk
Splashdown Water Birth Services – provides information and pool hire for women planning to labour in water

www.whattoexpect.com
What to Expect – general comprehensive pregnancy information

www.women-returners.co.uk
Women Returner's Network – advice, information, research and lobbying network for women returning to work after a break

www.womensaid.org.uk
Women's Aid (domestic violence)

www.workingfamilies.org.uk
Working Families – help to balance work and family life

Index

Page numbers in **_bold italic_** are for illustrations and diagrams; page numbers in **bold** are for glossary references

abbreviations, used in maternity notes, _19–22_

abdominal exercises, _238_

abnormalities, tests for, _67, 68, 69, 70_

acne, _71_

Aconite, 144

activities, _see_ exercise(s); recreational activities

acupressure wristbands, _76, 77, 168_

acupuncture points, _147, 157–8, 159, 162, 163_

acupuncture/acupressure, _76, 157–8_, **258**

AFP (alphfeto protein) test, _67_

afterbirth, _see_ placenta

alcohol
   in Bach flower remedies, _252_
   and diet, _57, 59, 60, 62, 66_
   and stress control, _24, 26_
   see also drugs; harmful stimulants; smoking

Alexander technique, _25_, **258**

allergies, 4

alphfeto protein (AFP) test, _67_

amniocentesis, _67_

anaemia, _60, 109, 110, 160_

anaesthetic, spinal, _140, 150–1, 166_

anaesthetists, _120_

anal intercourse, _39_

antenatal appointments, _17_
   see also maternity care

antenatal tests, _67–70_

anxiety, _140–1_
   see also emotions and feelings

APGAR score, _138, 150_

Apis, 90

arnica, _170, 227, 248_

aromatherapy, for
   backache, sciatica and pubic discomfort, _79_
   if Caesarean needed, _168–9_
   carpal tunnel syndrome, _90_
   constipation, _25, 229_
   contractions, _143_
   perineum care, _227_
   safe use of, _248–51_
   sleeping problems, _48_
   starting labour, _157_
   see also essential oils

artificial hormones, _137, 138, 155–6_

aspirin, _60, 61_

baby
   appearance at birth, _137_
   birth position, _132, 133, 155, 160–5_
   breathing at birth, _137, 138, 150_
   coping with crying, _213–16_
   impact on you as a couple, 6
   meeting and greeting, _177–9_
   packing items for birth, _106_
   size at birth, _132_
   suckling, _229–30, 234–5_
   unwise to use essential oils on, _248_
   see also breastfeeding

babysitters, _217_, **263**

Bach flower remedies, for
   breastfeeding, _233_
   if Caesarean needed, _169_
   contractions, _143_
   headaches, _88_
   perineum care, _227_
   pregnancy stress, _25_
   safe use of, _252–5_
   sex in pregnancy, _36_
   website, **263**

backache, *45, 49, 55, 77–80, 78–80, 135*

baking powder (sodium bicarbonate), *85*

balance, *see* work–life balance

bathing, and contractions, *146*

beauty tips, *70–4*

beds, and sleep, *49*

bedtime routines, *191–2, 208, 221*
  see also sleep

behaviour
  during labour, *136*
  sibling rivalry, *188–9*

benefits, social, *43–4, 126–7*

birth
  choosing birth place, *100–3, 161*
  due dates, *9, 154–5*
  emotions before and during, *97–9*
  as natural process, *156*
  planning for, *106–11*
  preparation for labour, *104–5*
  professional maternity carers, *117–23*
  as sexual experience, *115*
  see also contractions; labour; post-natal period

birth centres, *101–2*

birth companions, *103, 115–18, 121–3, 128–9, 142*

birth de-briefing, *185*

birth defects, and nutrition, *56*

birth notification cards, *106, 128, 205, 210*

birth plans, *106–7, 111*

Birth Support Therapists, *121–2*

birthing ball, *143*

birthing pools (water births), *108, 149, 152–3*

Bladder 67 point, *162, 163*

bleeding
  and delivery of placenta, *138, 141*
  implantation bleeding, *52*
  in newborn, *110*
  vaginal, after birth, *225*

blood
  circulation, *53–4, 170*
  clotting, *77, 252*

blood pressure
  high, *53, 87, 155*
  low, and epidurals, *150*

blood tests, *68, 69*

body
  baby's birth position, *132, 133, 155, 160–5*
  beauty tips, *70–4*
  changes in, *51–7, 195*
  posture and backache, *78–9*
  preparation for labour, *98*
  recovery after pregnancy and birth, *167–8, 191, 210, 224–8*
  sleeping positions, *49*
  see also physical well-being

bottle-feeding, *219–20, 231, 232–3*

bras, supportive, *53, 55, 78–9*

Braxton Hick contractions, *98, 133, 134*

breaks, *see* holidays and breaks; maternity leave and pay; relaxation

breastfeeding, *53, 110, 219–20, 229–36, 264*

breasts, *52–3, 55, 235–6*

breathing
  baby's, at birth, *137, 138, 150*
  during labour, *136, 137, 143*
  post-natal exercises, *227, 237*
  and visualization, *25–6*

breech presentation, *160–5*

bromelain, *160*

Caesarean sections, *157, 161, 162, 165–70*

caffeine, *56, 66*

Calcarea carb, *90*

calcium, *62*

cap (diaphragm), *194–5*

carbohydrates, *58*

cardiotocography (CTG), *68*

carers, *see* birth companions; health professionals; midwives

carpal tunnel syndrome, *89–91*

carrying and lifting, *78–9*

Caulophyllum, *144, 158*

Causticum, *86, 90*

cervix, *52, 133, 134, 136*

chamomile tea, *48, 90*

Chamomilla, *144, 158, 236*

child benefit, *43*
child tax credit, *43*
childcare, *219*
children
    present at birth, *116–17*
    responses to new baby, *188–9*
    responses to pregnancy, *32–3*
    see also relationships
Chinese medicine, *162*
chiropractic, *165*, *258–9*
chlamydia, *39*
chorionic villus (CVS), *68*
Cimicifuga, *144*, *158*
circulation, *see* bleeding; blood
Citizens Advice website, *43*, *262*
citrus oils, *229*, *249*, *251*
clothes
    for baby, *106*
    for labour and after birth,
        105, *143–4*
    maternity belts, *80*
    maternity bras, *53*, *55*, *78–9*
cobalamin (vitamin B$_{12}$), *60*
Cocculus, *76*
coffea, *48*
Colchium, *76*
colostrum, *53*
combined contraceptive pill (oral), *200*
companions, during labour and birth,
    103, *115–18*, *121–3*, *128–9*, *142*
complementary therapies, safe use of,
    245–57
    see also acupuncture;
        aromatherapy; Chinese medicine;
        chiropractic; homeopathic
        remedies; massage; reflexology;
        self-help techniques; t'ai chi
complementary therapists, *121–2*,
    122–3, *162*, *265*
complications, *6*, *153–4*, *155*
    Caesarean births, *162*, *166*, *167*
conception, *6–9*
condoms, *193–4*
constipation, *80–2*, *227–8*, *228–9*
contraception
    cap (diaphragm), *194–5*
    condoms, *193–4*
    implants, *198*

injections, *197–8*
IUDs (coils), *196–7*
natural family planning, *195–6*
oral (Pill), *3*, *60*, *61*, *199–200*
patches, *199*
and planning a pregnancy, *3*
sterilization, *201–2*
contractions, *98*, *108*, *132*, *139–42*
    Braxton Hick, *98*, *133*, *134*
    first stage, *135*, *136*
    second stage, *136–7*
    third stage, *109*, *137–8*
    working with, *143–6*
    see also birth; labour
cord, umbilical, *110*
cordocentesis, *68*
cortisol, *25*
counselling, *6*, *184–5*, *259*
cramp, *54*
craniosacral therapy, *259*
cravings, *54*
crying, *213–16*
CTG (cardiotocography), *68*
CVS (chorionic villus), *68*
cycling, *45*

dancing, *45*
date of birth, expected, *9*, *154–5*
dental care, *43*
depression, post-natal, *182*, *183–4*
diabetes, *28*, *69*, *265*
diaphragm (cap), *194–5*
diaries, *13–14*
diet, *55–62*
    balanced, *57*
    for breastfeeding, *233*
    and constipation, *81*
    and digestive system, *54*
    fluid intake, *57*, *64*, *81*, *233*
    foods to avoid, *65–7*
    and haemorrhoids, *83*
    harmful stimulants, *3–4*, *48*, *56*,
        66, *87*, *212*
    heartburn and indigestion, *85*
    and morning sickness, *75*
    preconception and conception,
        3–4
    relaxation and sleep, *48*, *212*

and safe use of homeopathic
remedies, 247
and skin care, 72
and weight gain, 63–4
and weight loss, 240
see also nutrition
disability living allowance, 43
diseases, *see* infections
doctors, 117, 118, 119–21
'doers' and 'feelers', 15, 23
doulas, 121–2
Down's syndrome, 70, 265
driving, posture for, 79
drugs
and complementary
treatments, 247, 252
for pain relief, 80, 87, 149–50
recreational, 4, 24, 56
to avoid, 61, 62, 65, 66–7, 252
see also alcohol; harmful
stimulants; smoking
dry skin, 71
due dates, 9, 154–5

eating
during labour, 108
and sleeping routines, 212
see also breastfeeding; diet;
nutrition
ECV (external cephalic version), 161–2
emotions and feelings, 11–29
asking for help, 13
before and during the birth, 97–9,
140–1
and choice of birth place,
100–3, 161
diary of, 13–14
difficult situations, 28, 29
first reactions to pregnancy, 11–12
maternity care, getting what you
would like, 16–18
maternity notes, abbreviations and
terms used, 18–23
partner's feelings, 5–6, 14–15,
35–7, 114, 128, 183
post-natal period, 177–9, 182–5
preparation for labour, 104–5
returning to work, 220–1, 222

sharing your feelings, 5–6, 15–16, 36
stress control, 23–7
towards baby's crying, 216
see also relationships; sexual
activity
endorphins, 35, 140
Entonox™, 148
epidurals, 140, 150–1, 166
epinephrine (adrenaline), 25
episiotomies, 109, 165, 192, 226
equipment, for labour/after birth,
105–6, 143–4
essential fatty acids, 58
essential oils, for
backache, sciatica and pubic
discomfort, 79
breastfeeding, 229
if Caesarean needed, 168–9
carpal tunnel syndrome, 90
headaches, 88
packing for labour, 105
perineum care, 227
pregnancy stress, 25
safe use of, 248–51
sex in pregnancy, 36
sleeping problems, 48
see also aromatherapy
examinations
post-natal, 191
vaginal, 107–8
exercise(s)
de-stress and relaxation, 26, 27,
87, 170
during pregnancy, 44–6
head and neck, 87
pelvic floor, 55, 170, 237
post-natal, 236–40, 268
expressing milk, 219–20
external cephalic version (ECV), 161–2
eyesight tests, 87

face, beauty care, 71
'facilitators' and 'regulators', 15, 23
families, *see* relationships
family planning, 190–3, 266
contraception, 193–202
fathers, *see* partners
fatty acids, essential, 58

feeding, *see* breastfeeding
'feel good' chemicals, *132, 140*
'feelers' and 'doers', *15, 23*
feelings, *see* emotions and feelings;
  relationships
feet
    and beauty care, *73–4*
    reflexology treatment, *90, 91*
female condoms, *194*
female sterilization, *201*
finances
    and choice of where to give
      birth, *103, 161*
    cost of essential oils, *249*
    and return to work, *218–19*
financial benefits, *43–4, 64*
fingernails, *73*
fitness, post-natal, *239–40*
    see also exercise(s); recreational
      activities
flexible working hours, *220*
fluid intake, *4, 57, 64, 81, 233*
fluid retention, *63, 164, 224*
folic acid, *56, 60*
food, *see* diet
forceps delivery, *165*
free birthing, *121*
friends, *211*
    see also mother and baby groups;
      relationships; visitors
fruit, *57*

Gall bladder 21 point, *159*
gas and air (nitrous oxide and
  oxygen), *148*
Gelsemium, *144*
general practitioners, *119–20*
German measles (rubella), *4*
ginger, *75, 77, 86, 169, 252*
glucose tolerance (GTT), *69*
GPs, *119–20*
grandparents, *187*
GTT (glucose tolerance), *69*
guilt, *220–1, 222*
gynaecologists, *119*

haemorrhage, *see* bleeding
haemorrhoids (piles), *39, 83–4*

hair, beauty care, *71–2*
hands, beauty care, *73–4*
harmful stimulants, *3–4, 48, 56, 66,*
  87, 212
    see also alcohol; drugs; smoking
hazardous substances, *4–5*
head and neck exercises, *87*
headaches, *86–8*
healing crisis, *247*
health, *see* diet; exercise(s); physical
  well-being
health professionals, *16–18, 117–23*
health visitors, *120*
heartburn (indigestion), *49, 84–6*
herbal medicines
    if Caesarean is needed, *169–70*
    for carpal tunnel syndrome, *90*
    for heartburn and indigestion, *86*
    safe use of, *251–2*
    see also homeopathic remedies
hereditary conditions, *6*
high blood pressure, *53, 87, 155*
high fibre foods, *81*
HIV, *39*
holidays and breaks, *41, 126–7*
home births, *100–1, 266*
home life, *see* work–life balance
homeopathic remedies, for
    breastfeeding problems, *236*
    breech position, *164–5*
    care of perineum, *227*
    carpal tunnel syndrome, *90*
    contractions, *144–5*
    haemorrhoids, *84*
    headaches, *88*
    heartburn and indigestion, *86*
    how to use safely, *246–8*
    induction, *158, 160*
    morning sickness, *76*
    pain relief, *80*
    sleeping problems, *48*
    see also self-help techniques
hormone injections, *137, 138*
hormones
    at conception, *8*
    during labour, *98, 139, 140–2*
    during pregnancy, *9, 52, 54, 80,*
      84, 140

during sex, *35, 139–40, 156*
'feel good' chemicals, *132, 140*
in post-natal period, *182–3, 229*
and stress control, *25, 142*
horse riding, *45*
hospital births, *100, 102–3*
hospital visitors, *209*
housework, *78, 205–7*
hygiene, personal, *225–6*
hypnosis, *26, 64*
hypnotherapy, *145, 165,* **259**

I don't know how she does it
(Pearson), *221–2*
implantation bleeding, *52*
indigestion (heartburn), *49, 84–6*
induction, *154–60*
infections
    sexually transmitted, *39*
    transmitted in hospitals, *209*
    urinary, *54, 225*
injections
    contraceptive, *197–8*
    hormone, *137, 138*
internal (vaginal) examinations,
107–8, 134
interventions, during birth, *103*
intrauterine contraceptive device
(coil), *196*
intrauterine system (Mirena™ coil), *197*
investigations, antenatal, *67–70*
Ipecacuanha, *76*
iron/iron tablets, *56, 62, 81*
IUD (coil), *196*

jacuzzis, *46*
juniper berry oil, *90*

labour, *131–9*
    aromatherapy use during, *250–1*
    and birth planning, *106–11, 126–8,*
    184–5
    body's preparation for, *98*
    breech presentation, *160–5*
    Caesarean sections, *157, 161, 162,*
    165–70
    complications, *153–4, 155, 162*
    contractions, *98, 108, 139–46*

conventional pain relief, *146–54*
    induction, *154–60*
    length of, *98–9, 138*
    preparation for, *104–6*
    rest, during and after, *126–8, 182–3*
    stages of, *134–5, 136–7, 137–8, 139*
    and water birth, *152–3*
    see also birth; contractions
lactation process, *229–30,* **230**
Large Intestine 4 point, *157,* **159**
lavender oil, for
    backache, sciatica and pubic
      discomfort, *79*
    if Caesarean needed, *168, 169*
    headaches, *88*
    perineum care, *227*
    safe use of, *249, 251*
    sleeping problems, *48*
leave, statutory maternity and
paternity, *44*
legal requirements, *117–18, 122, 135,*
139
length (time)
    of contractions, *135*
    of labour, *98–9, 138*
    of pregnancy, *9, 131*
    see also due dates; size; weight
      gain; weight loss
lifting and carrying, *78–9*
Lycopodium, *84, 90, 144*

make up, and beauty care, *71*
male condoms, *193*
male midwives, *117*
massage
    for backache, sciatica and pubic
      discomfort, *79*
    for breast massage, *235*
    if, Caesarean needed, *168–9*
    for constipation, *229*
    for contractions, *145*
    essential oils for, *249–50*
    for headaches, *88*
    nipple massage, *156*
    overview of, **259**
    for pregnancy stress, *26*
    for starting labour, *158*
masturbation, *39, 157*

maternity assistants, *120–1*
maternity belts, *80*
maternity benefits, *43–4*
maternity bras, *53, 55, 78–9*
maternity care, *16–18, 117–23*
    see also midwives
maternity grant, *44*
maternity leave and pay, *44, 179–80*
maternity notes, *18–23*
mattresses, *49*
medical conditions, *6, 69, 155*
medical staff, *16–18, 117–21*
medication, see drugs; prescription drugs
men, see male midwives; partners
menstrual cycle (periods), *7, 7, 8, 196*
mental adjustment, *132, 139, 140*
meptazinol, *149–50*
midwives, *117–18, 119, 135–6, 138–9, 185*
    see also maternity care
milk
    expressing, *219–20*
    leakages, *235–6*
    production, *229–30, 230*
    see also breastfeeding
mini pill (progesterone-only contraceptive pill), *199–200*
Mirena™ coil, *197*
miscarriage, and safe sex, *38*
mobility, during contractions, *145–6*
monitoring, during labour, *107*
mood swings, *24*
morning sickness, *60, 74–7, 252*
Morningwell™ audio CD, *76, 267*
morula, *8*
mother and baby groups, *211*
mothering role, planning for, *179–81*
mothers/mothers-in-law, *187–8*
movement, of baby, *55*
moxibustion, *162–4, 259*
mucus plug, *133, 134*

Natrum muriaticum, 86, 164
natural family planning, *195–6*
natural remedies, for
    if Caesarean is needed, *168–70*
    constipation, *82*
    haemorrhoids, *83–4*

headaches, *88*
heartburn and indigestion, *85*
how to use safely, *246*
morning sickness, *75–6, 252*
pain relief, *79–80, 88, 89–90*
see also complementary therapies; physical well-being; self-help techniques
neck and head exercises, *87*
NHS dental care, *43*
niacin (vitamin B$_3$), *59*
nipple massage, *156*
nipples, and breastfeeding, *234, 235*
nitrous oxide (laughing gas), *148*
noise, and sleep, *49*
norepinephrine, *25*
nuchal scan, *69*
nutrients, *58–62*
nutrition, *3–4, 26, 56–7*
    see also diet
Nux vomica, 76, 80, 84, 86, 164

obstetric ultrasonographer, *121*
obstetricians, *119*
occupational hazards, *5*
oestrogen, *229*
oral (combined) contraceptive pill, *3, 200*
oral sex, *39*
orgasms, *35, 156*
osteopathy, *260*
overdue labour, *131*
overeating, *64*
ovulation, *6–8*
oxytocin, *137, 139–40, 140–1*

paediatricians, *120*
pain
    during labour, *135, 137, 139, 140–1*
    during pregnancy, *45, 49, 55, 78–80*
    see also contractions
pain relief
    conventional, during labour, *142, 146–54*
    hormone response during labour, *140–1*
    natural remedies, *79–80, 88, 89–90*
    paracetamol, *80, 87*

papanicolaou (smear) test, 69
paracetamol, 80, 87
parenting
    'good enough' parents, 178
    grandparents, 187
    mothering, 179–81
    taking 'time out', 208, 209–10,
        216–18
part-time work, 218–19
partners (fathers)
    as birth companion, 116, 123,
        128–9
    and Caesarean births, 166–7
    delivery of baby, 118, 135
    feelings and emotions, 14–15,
        35–7, 114, 128, 183
    packing items for birth, 106
    paternity leave and pay, 44, 126–7
    rest and support during and after
        birth, 126–8, 182–3, 207
    sex during pregnancy, 34–9
    step-children's responses to
        pregnancy, 33
    time out with, 216–18
    website for, 265
    your relationship with, 5–6
    see also children; relationships
parturition, 131
    see also birth; labour
patch, contraceptive, 199
pay, maternity and paternity, 44, 126–7
Pearson, Alison, I don't know how she
    does it, 221–2
pelvic floor exercises, 55, 170, 237
pelvic girdle (symphysis pubis) pain, 45,
    49, 55, 77–80
pelvis, shape and size, 132
penetration
    post-natal sex, 192
    sex during pregnancy, 37, 38
peppermint, 75, 88
perineum, 137, 226–8
    see also episiotomies
periods (menstrual cycle), 7, 7, 8, 196
Persona™, 195
personal hygiene, 225–6
pethidine, 149, 150
pets, 33–4, 189–90

Phosophorus, 80
physical well-being, 51–94
    antenatal tests and
        investigations, 67–70
    backache, sciatica and pubis
        discomfort, 45, 49, 55, 78–80
    beauty tips, 70–4
    carpal tunnel syndrome, 89–91
    changes in your body, 51–7, 195
    constipation, 80–2, 227–8
    diet, 55–62
    drugs to avoid, 66–7
    foods to avoid, 65–7
    haemorrhoids (piles), 39, 83–4
    headaches, 86–8
    heartburn and indigestion, 84–6
    labour and birth, see child birth;
        contractions; labour
    morning sickness, 74–7, 252
    recovery from pregnancy and
        birth, 167–8, 191, 210, 224–8
    weight gain, 55, 63–4
    see also diet; exercise(s); nutrition
pigmentation, 72–3
piles (haemorrhoids), 39, 83–4
Pill (contraceptive), 3, 60, 61, 199–200
pillows, 49, 106
pineapple, 160
pituitary hormones, 8
placenta (afterbirth), 8, 9, 52
    delivery of, 109, 137–8, 141
plans/planning
    home life with a new baby,
        204–8
    labour and birth, 106–11, 126–8,
        184–5
    mothering role, 179–81
    for pregnancy, 3–6
    see also family planning; work–life
        balance
position
    birth, 132, 133, 155, 160–5
    for breastfeeding, 233–4
    for sex during pregnancy, 37
    sleeping positions, 49
    see also body; posture
positive thinking, 13, 64, 173, 221–2
post-natal 'blues', 182–3

post-natal period
    emotions and feelings, *177–9*,
      182–5
    examinations, *191*
    exercises and fitness, *227, 236–40,*
      268
    planning for mothering role,
      179–81
    self-care, *179–81, 207–8, 216–18*
    sexual activity, *191–2*
    support, *182–5, 187–8, 207–8,*
      209–11
    see also family planning; work–life
      balance
post-traumatic stress disorder (PTSD),
  184–5
postural therapies, *80*
posture
    backache, sciatica and pubic
      discomfort, *78–9*
    of mother during labour, *108*
    see also Alexander technique;
      body; position; t'ai chi; yoga
pre-eclampsia, *53, 87*
preconception, *3–6*
pregnancy diaries, *13–14*
premature labour, *131*
prescription drugs, *67*
professional maternity care, *16–18,*
  117–21
    semi-professional (doulas), *121–3*
progesterone, *54, 80, 84*
progesterone-only contraceptive pill
  (mini pill), *199–200*
prolactin, *229, 230*
prostaglandin, *156*
proteins, *58*
psychology, of pregnancy and birth,
  23, 182
PTSD (post-traumatic stress disorder),
  184–5
pubic discomfort, *45, 49, 55, 78–80*
Pulsatilla, for
    breastfeeding problems, *236*
    constipation, *82*
    contractions, *145*
    haemorrhoids, *84*
    heartburn, *86*

    morning sickness, *76*
    moxibustion, *164*
    starting labour, *158*
pyridoxine (vitamin B₆), *60*

Qi gong, *27,* **260**
questions, about maternity notes, *23*

raspberry leaf, *157, 160, 169, 251*
recreational activities, *217–18,*
  239–40
reflexology, *80, 88, 90, 158, 235,* **260**
'regulators' and 'facilitators', *15, 23*
relationships
    birth companions, *116–17, 123,*
      128–9
    family, *31–4, 187–90, 207*
    partners', *5–6, 34–9*
    siblings, *32, 188–9*
    see also emotions and feelings;
      partners; sexual activity;
      work–life balance
relaxation, *26–7, 48, 76, 87, 170*
reproductive organs, *52, 224–5*
Rescue remedy, *88, 169, 227, 233,*
  252–3
rest, *see* holidays and breaks;
  recreational activities; relaxation;
  sleep; 'time out'; work–life balance
rhythm method, *195–6*
riboflavin (vitamin B₂), *59*
routines, *191–2, 208, 212–13, 221*
rubella (German measles), *4*

safety
    at place of birth, *103*
    sex during pregnancy, *38–9*
    use of complementary therapies,
      245–6
St John's wort (*Hypericum*
  perforatum), *170*
saunas, *45–6*
scans, *9, 69, 70, 160–1*
sciatica, *45, 49, 55, 78–80*
self-care
    ante-natal, at work, *42*
    post-natal, *179–81, 207–8,*
      216–18

self-help techniques
  backache, sciatica and pubic
    discomfort, 79–80
  carpal tunnel syndrome, 89
  constipation, 228–9
  contractions, 143–6
  haemorrhoids, 83–4
  headaches, 88
  heartburn and indigestion, 85–6
  induction, 156–60
  morning sickness, 75–6, 252
  perineum, 226–8
  sore nipples, 235
  stress control, 25–7, 36, 48
  see also natural remedies; physical
    well-being
Sepia, 76, 80, 84, 146
sex (gender), of baby, 110
sexual activity
  best time for conception, 8
  birth as sexual experience, 115
  partners' relationships, 34–7,
    191–3
  post-natal, 191–2
  in pregnancy, 37–9
  and sleep, 48
  to encourage labour, 156–7
  see also relationships
sexually transmitted diseases, 39
shiatsu, 146, 147, 159, 260
'shows', 133, 134
siblings, 32, 188–9
  see also children; relationships
Sigh Out Slowly (SOS), 143
size
  and shape of baby, 155
  and shape of pelvis, 132
  see also due dates; length; weight
    gain; weight loss
skeleton, 55
skin, and beauty care, 71, 72–3
sleep
  after birth, 212–13
  bedtime routines, 191–2, 208, 221
  during pregnancy, 46–9
  and return to work, 220
sleeping positions, 49
smear (papanicolaou) test, 69

smoking, 24, 63, 64, 247
  websites, 262, 268
social contacts, see mother and baby
  groups; relationships; 'time out';
  visitors
Social Services, maternity benefits
  information, 43
sodium bicarbonate (baking powder), 85
SOS (Sigh Out Slowly), 143
sperm, 8
spinal anaesthetic, 140, 150–1, 166
Spleen 6 point, 158, 159
sports, to avoid during pregnancy, 45
  see also exercise(s)
stages of labour, 134–5, 136–7, 137–8,
  139
step-children, 33
sterilization, 201–2
stimulants, see alcohol; drugs; harmful
  stimulants; smoking
stitches, 192, 226, 248
  to close cervix, 38
  see also episiotomies
stress control, 23–5
  de-stressors, 25–7, 36, 48, 252
stress hormones, 25, 142, 165
stretch marks, 72
stretching exercises, 27
sun, protection from, 72–3
support
  during birth, 103, 115–23, 128–9,
    142
  financial, 43–4, 64
  post-natal, 182–5, 187–8, 207–8,
    209–11
  for special difficulties, 6, 29
  see also work–life balance
Sure Start, 64, 269
  maternity grant, 44
swimming, 27, 45
symphysis pubis (pelvic girdle) pain, 45,
  49, 55, 77–80

t'ai chi, 27, 260
tampons, 226
taste, sense of, 54
tax credit, 44
temperature, 46

TENS, 148–9, *149*, 263
tests, antenatal, 67–70
therapies, *see* natural remedies; physical well-being; self-help techniques
thiamin (vitamin B₁), 59
tiger balm, 88
time, *see* due dates; length
'time out', 208, 209–10, 216–18
tiredness, 47, 212
    see also bedtime routines; sleep
toddlers/young children, 32, 188
toilet habits, and constipation, 81
transition, 136
triple test, 69
twins/triplets, breech position, 160

UK
    breech births, 161
    maternity care, 16–18, 117–18, 122, 135, 139
    maternity unit visiting, 209
    paternity leave, 126–7
ultrasonographer, obstetric, 121
ultrasound scans, 9, 69, 70, 160–1
umbilical cord, 110
unassisted birthing, 122
unplanned pregnancy, 11–12
urinary infections, 225
urinary system, 54–5
USA
    maternity care, 118, 122
    paternity leave, 127
uterine muscle, 98, 132, 135, 157
    see also contractions
uterus, 8–9, 52, 132, 133

vaginal blood loss, 225
vaginal discharge
    during pregnancy, 52
    and sex during pregnancy, 35, 38
    'shows', 133, 134
vaginal (internal) examinations, 107–8
vaporizers, 25, 48, 250
vasectomy, 201
VBAC (vaginal birth after Caesarean), 167
vegetables, 57

ventouse extraction, 165
vibrators, *39*
visitors, 208–11
visualization, and breathing, 25–6
vitamins, 59–61, 110

water
    and healthy diet, 4, 57, 64, 81
    warm baths, 146
water births, 108, 149, 152–3, 269
waters breaking, 133, 135, 155
weight gain, 55, 63–4
weight loss, 237, 240
well-being, *see* physical well-being
work
    hazards at, 5
    maternity leave and pay, 44, 179–80
    mothering as 'new job', 179–81
    return to, 218–22, 269
    self-care at work, 42
    when to stop, 41–2
working environment, 42–3, 79
working tax credit, 44
work–life balance, 41–50, 204–22
    bedtime routines, 191–2, 208, 221
    before, during, after birth, 126–8, 177–85
    coping with crying baby, 213–16
    home life with new baby, 204–8
    maternity benefits, UK, 43–4
    meeting people/making friends, 211
    rest and sleep, 46–9, 212–13
    safe exercise, 44–6
    'time out', 208, 209–10, 216–18
    visitors, 208–10
    working during pregnancy, 41–2
    see also relationships

ylang ylang, 36, 79, 168, 249, 251
yoga, 27
young children/toddlers, 32, 188

zinc, 62